Praise for *One Ho*

"If you're a new mom, I highly recomm
Cox understands the challenges, frustrat
in trying to regain themselves after childbirth. I wish I had this book
years ago when I had my own children!"

— **Caroline Sutherland**, best-selling author of
The Body Knows . . . How to Stay Young

*"**One Hot Mama** is one hot, sanity-saving commodity for all*
moms of new babies everywhere! With grace, humor, and been-
there compassion, Erin Cox takes readers through the steps to renew
and invigorate their bodies, minds, and spirits after the life-altering
milestones of pregnancy and delivery. Never has a post-pregnancy
book been so thorough in addressing the genuine concerns and
vulnerabilities of a woman during this precious time in her life.
Erin's insights and encouragement will skyrocket the spirits of first-
time moms and seasoned pros alike, making them feel truly seen,
understood, and appreciated. I'll be gifting this one to every
pregnant woman I love!"

— **Lisa McCourt**, Joy Trainer and best-selling author of *Juicy Joy:*
7 Simple Steps to Your Glorious, Gutsy Self

"Erin Cox knows that the secret to being hot takes more than just a diet
and exercise book—it means getting in touch with your fire inside . . .
and this book shows you how to do that in the ultimate combination
of girlfriend, coach, and personal trainer. It may have taken 40 weeks
*to make a baby, but in just 12 weeks **One Hot Mama** can have people*
saying, 'Oh, Baby!' to the woman pushing the stroller."

— **Michelle Phillips**, TV and radio host, and best-selling
author of *The Beauty Blueprint: 8 Steps to Building the Life*
and Look of Your Dreams

ONE HOT MAMA

Hay House Titles of Related Interest

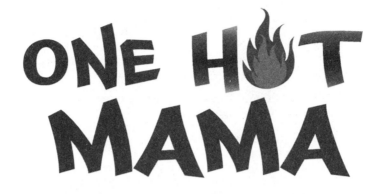

ONE H🔥T MAMA

The Guide to Getting Your Mind and Body Back After Baby

ERIN COX

HAY HOUSE, INC.
Carlsbad, California • New York City
London • Sydney • Johannesburg
Vancouver • Hong Kong • New Delhi

Published and distributed in the United States by: Hay House, Inc.: www.hay house.com® • *Published and distributed in Australia by:* Hay House Australia Pty. Ltd.: www.hayhouse.com.au • *Published and distributed in the United Kingdom by:* Hay House UK, Ltd.: www.hayhouse.co.uk • *Published and distributed in the Republic of South Africa by:* Hay House SA (Pty), Ltd.: www.hayhouse.co.za • *Distributed in Canada by:* Raincoast: www.raincoast.com • *Published in India by:* Hay House Publishers India: www.hayhouse.co.in

Cover design: Amy Rose Grigoriou • *Interior design:* Nick C. Welch
Interior photos: Peter Crouser Photography

Library of Congress Cataloging-in-Publication Data

Cox, Erin.
  One hot mama : the guide to getting your mind and body back after baby / Erin Cox. -- 1st ed.
    p. cm.
  ISBN 978-1-4019-3962-5 (tradepaper : alk. paper) 1. Motherhood--Psychological aspects. 2. Mothers--Health and hygiene. I. Title.
  HQ759.C78 2012
  306.874'3--dc23

                         2012022879

Tradepaper ISBN: 978-1-4019-3962-5
Digital ISBN: 978-1-4019-3963-2

15 14 13 12   4 3 2 1
1st edition, November 2012

Printed in the United States of America

SUSTAINABLE
FORESTRY
INITIATIVE

Certified Chain of Custody
Promoting Sustainable Forestry
www.sfiprogram.org
SFI-01268

SFI label applies to the text stock

*This book is dedicated to my very own hot mama,
Cindy Day, who has only become more fabulous
and fully herself with age. She raised me with love
and confidence to believe that I could do and achieve
anything. For this, I am ever grateful. My mom has
believed in me and supported me from the beginning.*

*This book is also dedicated to all the military spouses
around the world, who have taught me how to be
independent, gracious, and resilient while raising
children through all kinds of difficulties.*

CONTENTS

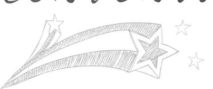

PREFACE

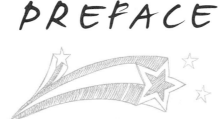

This book was written in my head long before it came to life on paper. Why? Because after I had my first baby, I searched for a book to help me pull myself back together—physically, intellectually, spiritually, and emotionally. But I was unable to find any resource that addressed my specific struggles, which so many other women I knew were also experiencing. Most new moms can't starve themselves like Hollywood actresses or follow standard dieting books. I definitely didn't find any books that discussed how to really be present and enjoy the experience of motherhood—or how to deal with mommy guilt or that feeling of wanting more. I was searching for inspiration. I wanted a realistic and sustainable way to lose the baby weight while being motivated to keep moving forward in my life. Since I couldn't find a book or program that addressed all of these imperative topics, I decided I would have to inspire myself.

At that time, I felt like I needed to express something beautiful that was trapped inside me, but it seemed like it was going to be impossible for a while, because I already felt overwhelmed by the duties of raising a new baby and working as an environmental consultant. When my first child was born, I was living at an extremely isolated Army post called Fort Irwin in the Mojave Desert—on a dead-end road, 40 miles from the nearest town. My husband, Steve, who is an Air Force F-15 pilot, was posted there to work as an air liaison officer with the Army for a few years.

Fort Irwin was like a fishbowl, where I could witness how women coped with motherhood while being cooped up in the middle of the desert. Oftentimes, they were raising children alone, with their husbands deployed for up to 15 months at a time. The entire neighborhood was developed around a park, where all the mothers hung out with their children every day. Even with a newborn, I sat there at the park with my stroller to get out and make new friends.

I observed mothers who were happy, kept themselves looking attractive, and seemed to thrive no matter what their circumstances were. I also met many moms who were frumpy, overweight, overwhelmed, and uninspired . . . they'd let themselves go. Their appearance reflected how they felt inside and what they thought about themselves. There seemed to be two distinct groups of women, and I could identify with both. I could see myself in every woman at that park. I realized that I was at a pivotal point in my life, having just had a baby. I could let myself go—or I could thrive, take really good care of myself, and still carry out my life's purpose. I knew which group of moms I strived to be like. I immediately began taking mental notes, developing a process for myself, and writing a guidebook in my head. I was then able to use the process with my second daughter three years later. Right after finishing this book, I will get to use the process with my third child, who will be a boy.

As a military spouse, I have moved four times in the past ten years. I've met women from all over the world, who have amazed me with the way they handle the demands of their daily lives while raising children. These women are incredibly independent and resilient, and they have inspired me and taught me so much. It is especially hard for military moms to carve out time for themselves and their careers, and many have sacrificed careers to follow their men—moving around the country and even across the world every two to three years! These women are thrust into new places and new climates, where they know no one, and have to nurture their children as they themselves are adjusting. Moving to a new place is always a little lonely at first.

Then they meet new friends from their new squadron, who come over to welcome them with dinner and a smile. They are invited out for coffee and play dates. They go to girls' nights out, and instant friendships form. Military friends become family, and these relationships span the miles and the years. I get tears in my eyes thinking of how many women and families, now spread around the world, that I truly love like flesh and blood.

I want to make you feel as though you are part of a very special "mom squadron." I want all women to know they are not alone and that there is someone out there who truly cares about them and wants them to succeed in their post-baby weight loss and in living a more joyful life. My mantra is that happy moms are the best moms. I want to support and nurture women when they are struggling with things we all struggle with—weight loss, time management, and carving out space for our creative endeavors.

I hope this book inspires you to set goals, learn useful tips, and maintain a positive attitude while achieving your ideal life. I am your biggest advocate and want to encourage you in any way I can.

For additional support, visit my website, **www.erincox.com**, for daily inspiration, healthy recipes, workouts, workshops, coaching, and other motivational ideas to keep you moving forward.

✦◻︎✦

Disclaimer: Before beginning the exercise program outlined in this book, please be sure to get the go-ahead from your physician. Most physicians recommend waiting to exercise for four to eight weeks postpartum, depending on the delivery. They also suggest starting slowly. Please be patient with your body and its abilities. Tailor the presented exercises and workout schedules to suit your limitations and fitness level. The activities recommended in this book are to be attempted at the reader's sole risk and discretion.

INTRODUCTION

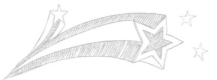

I am so excited that you have decided to join me on this journey to get your life back in gear and your body back in shape. Every mom I know wants to feel healthy, energetic, fulfilled, and beautiful. Raising needy little ones can make this more challenging; therefore, moms need an encouraging, empathetic, and supportive book to guide them on the course back to "themselves." What does it take to be one hot mama? Patience, self-care, self-love, and a lot of healthy eating and exercise.

One Hot Mama was written for moms by a mom who understands the challenges, frustrations, and hurdles women face in trying to regain themselves after childbirth. I came up with all of the ideas in this book as I recovered from my own pregnancies, so I completely understand what postpartum moms are feeling and experiencing each step along the way. The exercises and topics are presented at the appropriate challenge level as moms regain their physical and mental energy.

You may have recently given birth to your first baby or to your fourth. You might be six weeks postpartum, or maybe it's been two years since your child was born. This book is ideal for any woman who has recovered from delivery and needs a little inspiration and motivation to get her "self" back mentally, physically, and spiritually. I have developed a program based on my own experiences and those of dozens of fabulous moms. This program promises to make your life more fulfilling than it has ever been—while you enjoy the experience of motherhood fully. My main goal in writing this book is to offer you loving, supportive, and motivating guidance through a realistic and clear process that is completely doable for any woman. Please feel free to modify this program to suit your current mind-set and physical abilities.

Are You Ready to Get Back in Shape?

You will have the greatest success with this book if you are really ready for it, both physically and mentally. Take the first weeks postpartum to focus on bonding with your sweet baby and getting the sleep required to simply sustain yourself and start your life as a mother off right! You will recover more fully and quickly if you concentrate on resting and recovering during those first weeks.

Also, be sure to wait until after you've had your six-week postpartum doctor's appointment and gotten the go-ahead to resume physical activity. I know that by about three weeks after having my second child, I was antsy; I got out and walked slowly with the stroller because my recovery was going so well. But it's important to take things very slowly, because your body is still healing and recovering. Five weeks after my first delivery, I went for a strenuous hike and ended up at the doctor's office with heavy bleeding. Start by going for leisurely walks and stretching. When your body feels really good doing these light activities and your doctor says go for it, you are physically ready to get started.

Psychologically, there comes a point when you are simply ready to reengage with the bigger world. Your days at home with a newborn are beautiful, but your brain simply wants to be challenged. When you start longing for something a little more, then you are at exactly the right place to start this program mentally. If you are feeling a little stir-crazy—as though you have a lot more to offer the world—then I am so excited to be your partner in helping you become clear on what the next phase of your life holds and how you can live each day with more joy.

Ways You Can Use This Book

This book is structured into 12 weeks (3 months), with each chapter representing one week. I personally enjoy following a structured plan, and I tried to make each week's reading just enough for you to digest without feeling overwhelming.

While the book is formatted this way, *you do not have to use the book this way.* I want you to go at your own pace. If you would like to spend two or three weeks on each chapter, please do so. Some chapters might be just right for you to complete in one week, while you might need more time for other chapters. There are no rules, and this book supports you in whatever pacing works best for you.

The weekly chapters have a consistent format. Each chapter starts with a timely topic, which is presented with personal stories, suggestions, and thought-provoking action items. In the "Nourishment" section, you will learn about proper nutrition, eating to sustain your energy level, and adopting healthy eating as a lifestyle rather than as a temporary diet plan.

Exercising is one of the key ingredients to losing post-baby pounds, which is why the "Fitness" section of each chapter contains fun and practical workout ideas, routines, and schedules to motivate you to get out there and discover how great it feels to exercise. The approach is practical and encouraging, keeping in mind that it can be painful to get back in shape, especially when you may already feel exhausted. The weekly workout schedules get progressively more demanding as you go through the book and get in better shape. Some weeks you might be able to fit in every workout, while other weeks you might not be able to do so for any number of reasons. Have a little compassion for yourself. Always do the best you can, and don't beat yourself up if you miss a workout or two.

This book considers the emotional as well as the physiological challenges of losing weight. Accordingly, each chapter features timely advice and self-care tips in the "Sanity Saver" section. These take-home ideas are easy actions that will make your life more relaxing and enjoyable while raising babies. Finally, each chapter closes with an "Affirmation for the Week" for you to read out loud or in your head to reaffirm everything you have just learned.

Setting Goals

If losing weight is your primary purpose for reading this book, I urge you to set a realistic and attainable weight-loss goal for yourself. Having a goal is important for achieving the greatest success. Remember that healthy, sustainable weight loss doesn't happen overnight, and it's safest to lose one to three pounds per week. Maybe your goal is simply to become a happier and more joyful mother, and that's perfectly fabulous as well.

Take the time now to fill in the primary goals you want to accomplish while reading this book. Refer back to them later to remind yourself why you are here! It might also be useful to track your weight once a week after the first full month to monitor your progress and see how your hard work is paying off.

What You Will Need

To help you get ready to start exercising and working out, I suggest you look through your drawers to make sure you have plenty of **comfortable workout clothes** and **supportive bras**.

As far as exercise equipment, I recommend having **two sets of dumbbells**, one lighter and one heavier. I have five-, eight-, and ten-pound dumbbells, which cover just about every exercise I want to do at home. If you have not lifted weights in over a year, start light, using three- and five-pound weights.

One of the workouts in the book features an **exercise ball.** I think an exercise ball is one of the best things a new mother can own. In addition to using the ball as an exercise tool, you can rock and bounce a fussy baby on it or lie on it to stretch your back and chest when you are tight from holding and feeding the baby. Inexpensive dumbbell weights and exercise balls can be found at any discount store, such as Target, or at any large sporting goods store. You will be glad to have these items at home, if you don't already!

I also suggest having a way to listen to music while you are exercising. I use my iPhone, but many people like iPods or other MP3 players. Listening to interesting podcasts or upbeat music makes workouts more pleasurable! There are some fantastic playlists on my website, **www.erincox.com.**

I discuss journaling in a few places in *One Hot Mama.* It would be a great idea to get a **beautiful journal** or some type of book to write in. Even if you don't consider yourself a writer in any way, I believe writing is an important tool for helping you become clear on many things in your life. The numerous benefits of writing down your thoughts, feelings, and goals are described in the book.

Finally, you will need to put lots of **fresh, healthy foods** on your grocery shopping list. As you go through this process, you will be motivated to eat healthier, less-processed food. While at the store, pick up a few inspirational magazines that feature nutritious recipes, exercises, or mindful-living ideas to help encourage you along the way! You can also visit my website for numerous recipes, the monthly workout schedule in an easy-to-print format, and other awesome free resources.

Are you ready to channel your inner hot mama? Turn the page, and let's get started on reinvigorating your life, restoring your mind, and reshaping your body!

★◻★

MONTH ONE

In the first month of this process, I urge you to practice a lot of self-love and patience. This is a time of major change in your life. I will help you learn how to take really good care of yourself and to rest when you need to, so you will have enough energy to start exercising regularly while caring for your family's needs. We will also discuss financial issues, which can be in a state of flux when a new baby arrives. In addition, we will focus on self-worth, your own progress, and not comparing your body or life to anyone else's. Finally, we will discuss getting into the rhythm of motherhood and how to enjoy your life to the fullest as you embark on this fabulous new adventure.

★▢★

Putting Yourself First

"Moms need to build up their strength and care for themselves first, when they can, so they have the energy and love to nurture their families."

— ERIN COX

Have you ever gotten to the end of your day and literally collapsed on the couch in exhaustion? Have you wondered if you will ever feel completely rested and energized again? Has your libido dropped to the point where you can't remember the last time you thought about sex? I think most moms have been there!

Mothers are instinctively programmed to make sure everyone's needs are met, often at the expense of meeting their own basic needs. When you're not getting enough rest or taking time for yourself, how can you expect to give your best to your children or have anything left over for connecting with your partner at the end of the day? How about sex?

When there are helpless babies and children who need to be fed and bathed, of course their needs are a priority. But all the other demands on your time and energy can be reorganized to make sure you can practice self-care—so you will have the energy to maintain the pace of your life, and do so with joy, presence, and peace.

Do you take time to nurture yourself by listening to what your body and soul need? Do you give yourself the time to rest when you need to? Do you set aside the time required to cultivate your dreams? I promise you that if you make yourself a priority at every opportunity, you will have more liveliness and love to give your family. Think about how refreshed you feel after a few hours alone, doing something you enjoy. Here is a recent comment from one of my girlfriends who is the stay-at-home mom of two young children: "I never thought sitting in a quiet, smelly oil-change waiting room could be as therapeutic as a spa service, but right now it's ranking high on relaxation." This cracked me up, but we've got to take a restful moment where we can get it, right?

Do you take time for self-care? By self-care, I mean caring for yourself physically, mentally, and spiritually. Are you taking the time to read books and learn new things? Are you getting the exercise you need to feel fit and have a healthy heart? Are you paying attention to the food you put in your mouth, ensuring that the majority of it goes to nourishing your body and making you feel magnificent? Do you make getting a good night's sleep a priority when you can? Do you take time to connect to a higher power and express gratitude through meditation or prayer?

If not, don't worry, because one of the purposes of this book is to help you find ways to carve time out of your hectic schedule to put yourself first. Babies require a lot of time and energy, but there are countless ways to keep them occupied. There are other great resources, such as babysitters, mother's-day-out programs, and childcare swapping, to allow you to pursue your passions and make sure you are well rested, centered, and healthy.

This week's chapter will offer you many road-tested methods for losing your baby weight, fitting in your workouts, getting more rest, and cultivating joy on a daily basis by taking time for simple pleasures. You will find numerous easy self-care suggestions ranging from taking a candlelit bath, indulging in dark chocolate and a glass of wine, and making sure you get enough sleep.

Is It Safe to Drink While Breastfeeding?

This is personal decision, but all the research I've done indicates that drinking an occasional glass or two of wine will not harm your baby while you are nursing. Here are a few pieces of information to help you make your own decision.

Alcohol in the bloodstream passes rather quickly into the milk, with peak levels occurring 30 to 60 minutes after drinking when drinking on an empty stomach and 60 to 90 minutes when drinking on a full stomach. Levels of alcohol are metabolized and leave your milk at the same rate.[1]

Less than 2 percent of the alcohol dose consumed by a nursing mother reaches her milk and blood.[2]

Alcohol is not stored in your breast milk and is metabolized at the same rate as in your blood and body. Therefore, there is no need to "pump and dump" unless you are away from your baby and need to pump for relief.

Most experts advise waiting two to three hours after drinking to nurse your baby and to limit your intake to one or two drinks.

The bottom line: Listen to your intuition, and have a drink or two occasionally, if you enjoy it. Just try to time your consumption of alcohol so that you won't need to feed your baby for a few hours.

Hot Mamas Take Care of Themselves

Your own happiness and well-being can feel quite secondary when you've got a new baby, but there is no better time to practice self-care and put your needs first (when you have the opportunity, of course). Self-care may involve something as simple as taking a few extra minutes to make yourself feel cute in the morning.

Feel Pretty

In addition to getting some rest, new moms need to do what they can to start feeling like themselves again. Get out of your sweats or pajamas! Take a bath or shower, and put on a little makeup! This is one of the most important tips for any new mom. It is so tempting to just stay in your comfy pajamas or sweats all day and night, but trust me on this one: You need to shower and get dressed every day if you possibly can. This is high on the recommendations lists of all of my girlfriends! Staying home in your sloppy clothes will make you feel even frumpier, more tired, and less put-together than you already do.

I remember looking in the mirror some mornings after what felt like a few minutes of sleep and thinking, *Who is that tired, old-looking woman?* The process of taking a hot shower and getting myself ready was like resuscitation; it brought me back to life each morning. The difference in the way I looked and felt before and after my shower was amazing. People who stopped by to meet my daughter would comment that I looked well rested and must be getting lots of sleep—but in reality, it was the daily shower, decent clothes, makeup, and hair brushing that kept me pulled together. This task was definitely easier on some days than others. Sometimes the daily shower didn't happen until my husband came home for lunch; and of course, on some days I just couldn't get it in, period. There was definitely a difference in my well-being and attitude on the days when I didn't get myself showered, dressed, and ready.

When possible, wake up before your baby and get in the shower, even if you just went to bed a few hours earlier. You can even fit this in during the day's first naptime. Stand there, take deep breaths, and just let the hot water relax and rejuvenate you. Think of your shower as a few precious minutes to yourself to feel human again. Wash the spit-up from your skin and the sleep from your eyes. I know you probably never thought showering in your own bathroom could be a spa-like experience, but compared to the grueling routine of being a new mom, it suddenly can be! Get yourself two types of body washes, one relaxing and one invigorating, and use whichever seems more appropriate at the time.

After your shower, you don't have to spend a long time getting ready. In all likelihood, you won't have more than a few minutes. If you've got to put on maternity or bigger jeans, so be it. Otherwise, slip into some comfy yoga-type pants and a nice clean shirt, and you will feel great. Nobody expects a new mom to wear an awesome, stylish outfit at this point, but dress in something that makes you feel as good as possible, for your own sake!

After a few weeks at home, I was ready for some real pants. I couldn't stand another day in my maternity clothes. It was a mental thing that was hard for me to overcome, but I went out and bought some jeans and nice pants that were two sizes larger than normal. In my pre-baby delusion, I had assumed I'd go from maternity jeans right back to my regular size within a few weeks. Not quite! Now, I do hear of women from time to time who can actually pull this off. For example, I have a new friend in her mid-30s who wore her regular jeans within a week of delivering her fourth child! She is a freak of nature, based on the hundreds of moms I have known. I know of a young mother who was in her early 20s when she delivered her first child; she was back to her regular weight within weeks. There are certainly some benefits to being a young mom, and the possibility that you might fit into your regular jeans when you get home from the hospital could be a reality for you. For the rest of us, get real and buy some attractive jeans in a bigger size! Just know in the back of your mind that these are temporary and simply serve to make you feel comfortable and look cute in the short term.

There are great makeup sticks and powder makeup compacts that can cover under-eye bags and blotchy skin in a matter of seconds. My favorite is a foundation stick by Bobbi Brown. Add a little blush, mascara, and lipstick or gloss and you will look much less like a haggard, sleepless old mom and more like the put-together, hot woman you truly are.

Be Kind and Gentle with Yourself

If you are feeling uncomfortable and exhausted, it may be difficult to trust your instincts in mothering your often-finicky, screaming new baby. Whenever things weren't going so smoothly with feeding or getting the baby to sleep, I tended to question my ability to be a good mother to my helpless child. It was so easy in my overtired and foggy state to be really hard on myself and even my husband. Be kind to yourself, and know you're a good mother. Give your body (and your partner) a break, too. Simply do the best you can in every moment.

Take a minute to really reflect on what your body's just done. In a matter of nine months, you have grown a human being from two cells. You have accommodated another life within your womb. You have nourished and protected this life, and your body has known what to do every step of the way. Think of yourself as a maternal goddess, because you have really gone through something quite magical. Accept that your body is a bit stretched out of shape, but don't dwell on that. I know it's a cliché, but your body took nine months to grow to that size to accommodate the developing baby, so how can you expect it to go back to normal much more quickly? Be kind to yourself; your body is amazing.

An important way to treat yourself kindly is to hide your scale for a few more weeks! You may have weighed yourself as a starting point when you set your weight-loss goals, but put the scale away for now. If you do step on the scale for the sake of curiosity, I forewarn you that you may not like what you see. My advice is to skip the scale altogether during the first month of this plan. You can get excited to start watching the pounds drop as you weigh yourself once per week during the second and third months.

Be a Little Selfish

Something happens to women the moment we become mothers, and we instantly start putting everyone and everything before ourselves. Women have a tendency to work toward the greater good at all times, but this is intensified once we have babies. When I say to be a little selfish, I really mean for you to preserve and protect your energy, mind, body, and spirit. Selfish isn't always a bad thing.

New babies need so much. I felt like the life was being sucked out of me on some days! Babies require what feels like constant feeding, changing, rocking, cuddling, etc. We give so much for these babies—our bodies, breasts, beauty, sanity . . . at least it feels that way sometimes. Just like a baby needs so much for survival, a mother needs support so she can keep going.

When someone offers to bring you a meal, accept it with love and gratitude. When another friend offers to drive your older children to and from preschool, let her! When your mom wants to do all of your laundry, allow her to do it. When your husband gets up in the middle of the night to calm your crying baby, bless him. People want to give, and after you have a baby is a time when you should accept. Be a little selfish. The word *selfish* has a negative connotation. But in this situation, it means looking out for yourself so you have something left to give your baby, who needs so much of you. It's your time to accept the kindness of friends and family with appreciation.

Watch Out for Hormones!

You will probably find yourself feeling irritable, overwhelmed, anxious, and even weepy at times during your first months as a mom. On top of the sleep deprivation and caring for a very needy baby, you've got crazy hormone fluctuations, too!

Have you found yourself tearing up when gazing in disbelief at your baby, who is asleep in your arms? I fought the urge to weep at anything remotely touching on TV or a sweet note written in a card to me. Something akin to this happens to most new moms regularly, and for some moms, this is the extent of the baby blues. If you're feeling something more serious and have thoughts of harming your baby or yourself, put down this book and call your obstetrician immediately to discuss your thoughts and feelings.

My mom came to stay for a few weeks after my first child was born. With her there to help, I was doing pretty well. I got my daily showers in, I didn't worry much about cooking or cleaning, I had the comic relief and unwavering support of my mom, and when I needed a nap, I passed my baby off to willing and loving arms. I was scared to death for my mom to go home. Could we do it without her? I'd really come to depend on her for cheeriness, advice, housekeeping, cooking, and baby holding.

The morning after Mom left, my husband, Steve, got up, showered, put on his flight suit, and went back to work. I was home alone with the baby for the first time. Quietness and spending a lot of time without another adult around can force one to deal with the reality of the present moment. We had been visiting, entertaining, doing, and going since I had come home from the hospital so much that things hadn't really sunk in. The weight and magnitude of how much my life had changed was finally real, and this first day alone was a reality check. I was scared, lonely, tired, and overwhelmed. My hormones were raging and a bit crazy, and my ranting inner dialogue went something like this as my husband drove away:

> *His good-bye kiss was kind of quick and cold, which tells me that he's excited to go back to work and get out of here. How could he leave me alone? That jerk. How is this fair, that he gets to drive away in his car by himself with a mug of coffee like a real adult and go to work like nothing's changed for him, while I'm here and I'm fat and my boobs hurt and I'm sore and—oh God—in another few minutes I'm going to have to try to feed my little eel with my bleeding nipples and I don't think I can do it? I am lonely, and I can't call my mom because she will worry herself sick about me. I can't let anyone else know I am not thrilled when I have such a perfect new baby.*

Finally, I broke down in tears. Then I took a deep breath. And another deep breath. I reassured myself that I could do anything, and I reminded myself of my wonderful family and dozens of awesome friends who were sending me love. Honestly, it helped. My deep breaths became my meditation and brought me peace during this time.

The men in our lives can be a bit confused by our craziness during this time. You know in the rational part of your brain that you shouldn't be upset about certain things, but you are. I took it personally that my husband seemed a little excited about going back to work, as if it was a choice for him to leave me alone. You, too, might want to cry as your partner leaves you alone with the baby (and possibly other needy children) and gets to act like a "real" adult and have intellectual conversations with other adults throughout the day. You might be back at work yourself, having those adult interactions all day, but also realizing that it's not always glamorous and wonderful to have to get up and leave a new baby every morning. Like my husband, however, working moms know there is some peace and relief to be able to get up, get dressed, and get out of the house. For now, if you're home with the baby, feeling fat, sloppy, alone, exhausted, and weepy, know that this mind play is caused by crazy hormones, with a little extreme exhaustion thrown in.

If and when you are feeling especially down, just take a deep breath, experience your tears and frustration fully, and know and believe that it's just the hormones taking over your thoughts. If you are a praying person, pray for strength; if you meditate, be still with God and breathe; or simply breathe if that's all you can do. You may have to reaffirm that you are okay and doing great each and every morning (or every hour for that matter). But know that slowly your hormones will readjust themselves, you will start getting more sleep, and you will feel more and more like yourself with each passing day. Whenever I couldn't get the baby to stop crying or the pain of latching on was excruciating, I'd try to become conscious, relax, and focus on a few deep breaths. The negative fog would lift—for the moment anyway. Each time I breathed through a difficult moment, it got easier, and my confidence in myself as a mother grew.

The powerful effect of raging hormones on your mood and thought patterns should not be understated. It takes mental strength to overcome the negative thought patterns that can fill your mind when your body is so chemically confused and exhausted. If you are unable to overcome negativity and the sense of being overwhelmed, try to step back in your mind and observe your thoughts. I learned to do this, and it helped me realize when I was being completely irrational. I'd say or think something pretty terrible, and then I'd pause to wonder where the heck it came from. Being more aware and present in every moment helped me to observe my thoughts and feelings before "shooting off the cuff." This practice reduced fighting and tension, and actually caused me to laugh at myself sometimes. I was being a crazy lady!

Try to observe your feelings and thoughts as though you were a bystander in your own brain. The real you is inside but is just temporarily overtaken by hormone-driven thoughts. Eckhart Tolle calls these superficial thoughts, or mind chatter—your ego—while your presence beneath it all is the real you. Don't worry; the joyous, fun, collected, rational woman you really are is still within you, and she will return (mostly) full-time very soon, if she hasn't already.

The Four Keys to Weight Loss

After giving birth the first time, I remember looking down at an unrecognizable body, wondering how it could ever be back to "normal" again. The swelling, rolls, and loose skin on my belly literally made me feel sick, and I looked at myself with disgust. I was scared. By patiently taking care of myself, getting enough rest, eating mostly healthy foods, and exercising a lot, I slowly lost all the weight. My second and third pregnancies didn't scare me because I'd gained upwards of 40 pounds in my previous pregnancies and lost it all each time. I knew I could do it. You can do it, too.

From my own experiences and those of my girlfriends and from years of observation and tons of research, I have concluded that there are four pieces to the weight loss puzzle. If you put all four of them together, you are sure to get your best body back for good.

Adequate Sleep + Healthy Eating + Exercise + Body Love
= Weight Loss

Most weight loss programs focus on one or maybe two of these pieces, but to get to your healthy, ideal weight and stay there, all four of these elements should be present in your life. You can lose weight by implementing one or two of the components, but it takes so much more effort and is more difficult to sustain long-term.

This four-pronged approach is more of a lifestyle, so you will never feel deprived or as though you are "on a diet."

Psychologically, I believe that when you tell yourself you're on a diet, you are telling yourself that you are not okay or good enough the way you are, so you are going to deprive yourself to get to whatever your idea of skinny is. Rather, if your mind-set is that you are eating well and exercising so that your body feels great, you have energy, and your outside reflects the beauty inside, then weight loss becomes an act of self-love.

This book will cover the four keys to weight loss in detail, starting with the one I believe new mothers need the most: sleep.

Key One for Weight Loss Is Adequate Sleep

Losing weight will be significantly more difficult if you aren't getting enough rest. Research shows a direct correlation between the amount of sleep you get and your weight. *The Journal of the American Medical Association* and *The Lancet* have both published academic research indicating that sleep loss increases hunger and affects the body's metabolism, making it more difficult to maintain or lose weight.[3, 4]

There are numerous ugly side effects of sleep loss that make it harder for mothers of new babies to lose weight. Additionally, when we are exhausted from insufficient sleep, we are not able to learn or remember as well, and our brains simply don't function like they should. Finally, a lack of sleep is linked to depression and feeling more emotional and overwhelmed.

Moms of Young Children = Exhaustion

It seems unfair that the time in your life when you want to lose weight the most, your often-sleepless circumstances make it that much more difficult to do so. Nurturing a baby is one of the most enriching, fabulous, and amazing things you will ever do; at times, it will also be one of the most trying, tiring, and difficult.

To be completely frank, the whole motherhood experience starts out with complete exhaustion. Do not underestimate the severe (but not permanent) impacts of sleep deprivation. After giving birth, your body is in the recovery process for months, so while your body is trying to heal and recover, you are also usually in one of the most sleep-deprived conditions of your life.

I remember looking in the mirror after a particularly rough night and feeling as though I had aged a decade overnight. When speaking, I'd lose my train of thought mid-sentence. My husband would look at me with horror, secretly hoping his once-eloquent and smart wife hadn't disappeared forever. It's a kind of tired that you just can't understand until you experience it. Being awakened numerous times throughout the night for weeks—and often months—on end can create a woman that you hardly recognize. The amazing thing is that many of us become accustomed to being in a foggy, sleepy state; it simply becomes our new reality. And then, we slowly reemerge as our babies start to sleep. The sooner we can get to this phase, the better.

When my first child was a few weeks old, I remember a "wake up every hour" kind of night when I could not get her to stop screaming. It was a gut-wrenching, shrill newborn scream, intended to fill your brain with so much noise that you can do nothing else but pay attention! The utter exhaustion felt like a heavy blanket draped over me, and my nerves were as raw as a freshly gaping wound. I felt nauseous from such a strong desire to pass out. I remember holding the baby in my arms, and all of a sudden, I had a nearly uncontrollable urge to squeeze her or shake her or do anything I had to get her to stop crying—so I could finally sleep. Instead of squeezing my baby, I ended up yelling to release some of the frustration and tension. That actually shocked her quiet for a few minutes!

The next morning, I remembered with disgust the way I had nearly lost control of myself. My husband is a military aviator, and getting sleep is a matter of life and death for him, so I took sole responsibility for waking up with the baby during the week. My near-breakdown let me know that I desperately needed to get some rest. My body felt like it was literally breaking down. That Saturday night, I set my husband up with bottles and the baby monitor an inch from his head on full blast. Then I settled into our guest room with earplugs and a pillow over my head. I woke up seven hours later, breasts ready to explode, but feeling sharp, rested, and as though I could carry on an intelligent conversation. I even felt as though I might have the energy to go for a run.

The Saturday-night sleep became my saving grace—a real turning point in motherhood for me. I became a sleep hoarder for the first time in my life. I suggest that you, too, become a sleep hoarder. Take every opportunity to rest, and do everything you can to get at least 7 or 8 hours of sleep during every 24-hour period.

Getting adequate sleep is one of the first steps that will help you feel like yourself again. Your appetite will regulate itself because you won't need to eat to get an energy boost. The neurons in your brain will fire, and you will start being able to clearly convey the thoughts in your head. Your emotions will begin to regulate. Your postpartum mood swings will start to swing smaller and smaller, until your mental state is as smooth and peaceful as a glassy pond.

I want to emphasize that I wrote this section as much for myself as for all of you. I know how difficult it is to get enough rest—and how I tend to want to work on my computer or clean the house rather than nap with my babies. My research has persuaded me to do what I can to get more sleep, and the impacts have been very noticeable and compelling.

Sleep Deprivation Impairs Your Ability to Lose Weight

Research has shown without a doubt that inadequate sleep dramatically affects our metabolism and makes it that much more difficult to lose weight. Namely, inadequate rest makes you hungry even when your body has had enough food. In addition, losing deep sleep leads to increases in fat storage.

Increased Hunger

Your body produces two hormones to help regulate your appetite: ghrelin and leptin. When you do not get enough sleep and rest, two things happen: First, levels of ghrelin increase, intensifying feelings of hunger. Second, levels of leptin decrease. Leptin is the hormone that makes you feel satisfied when eating, so without enough leptin, you will not feel as full after a normal-sized meal; hence, you will probably end up eating more.

Not only does sleep deprivation produce abnormal levels of ghrelin and leptin, but it also causes concentrations of the stress hormone cortisol to escalate in your body. When your body thinks it's under stress, your metabolism slows down and starts to crave calorie-dense comfort foods to help you survive the "tough times."

Increased Fat Storage

As if gaining 20 to 60 pounds to create a baby wasn't enough of a body-image killer, the resulting sleep deprivation interferes with the body's metabolism of carbohydrates—leading to elevated blood sugar and the storage of excess body fat. Elevated blood sugar will cause your body to produce too much insulin, which can induce insulin resistance and eventually lead to the development of diabetes.

Mothers of babies and small children often have interruptions in the deep-sleep phase, a crucial stage of sleep for hormone regulation. During the deep-sleep phase, your body secretes growth hormone (GH). Sleep deprivation will cause a significant decrease in your body's GH levels. Growth hormone has many remarkable properties: It stimulates cellular growth, reproduction, and regeneration; breaks down fat; increases muscle mass; strengthens bones; and boosts the immune system. A deficiency in GH can cause an increase in fat accumulation, a decrease in muscle tissue, and a decline in energy levels. Growth hormone is also said to improve the skin's tone and texture and reduce the effects of aging.

Therefore, a loss of deep sleep in mothers can lead to two things we want the very least: difficulty losing weight and a substantial decline in energy levels. Studies have shown that just one week of sleep deprivation will lead to significant decreases in GH levels in healthy adults.[5] This fact makes me want to go curl up in bed right now! Clearly, adequate sleep is a crucial component of weight loss.

Sleep Deprivation Impairs Your Brain

Sleep is crucial for repairing and regenerating our bodies, especially our brains, so we are able to function optimally. Sleep helps us to have sharp brains, enabling us to learn new things and perform better overall. When we don't get enough sleep, our brains can really suffer. Thinking, learning, and memory are dramatically impacted by sleep deprivation. When we aren't getting enough sleep, we experience impaired speech skills, a lack of creative thinking, and a reduced ability to multitask.

Thinking, Learning, and Memory

Research has repeatedly shown that the brain commits new facts, information, and experiences to memory during sleep through a procedure called memory consolidation. Not getting enough sleep makes it difficult to incorporate new information and learn new things. Yikes!

One of the ironic side effects of sleep deprivation is that we are no longer able to recognize how sleep deprived we are. We may feel only somewhat tired, but tests show that we have slower reaction times, weakened memory, and additional thinking impairments.[6] Studies consistently illustrate that even missing an hour or two of sleep can have devastating results. Most moms often miss an hour or two of sleep a night (or even three or four hours) for weeks on end. We need to do everything we can to make up for this deprivation.

Speech, Creative Thinking, and Multitasking

The functions of our brain's frontal lobe include speech, imagination, and creative thinking. This part of the brain is markedly impacted by a lack of sleep. People subjected to sleep deprivation in a study were less able to think imaginatively; they used clichés and unoriginal, repetitive phrases during creative writing exercises. These sleep-deprived subjects were also less eloquent and were unable to speak clearly; in some extreme cases, they exhibited slurred and slowed speech, as well as stuttering.[7]

All moms have to multitask at times, and inadequate sleep can reduce our ability to focus on several tasks at once. This impairment includes both the speed and the efficiency with which tasks can be completed.

Sleep Deprivation Can Make Us Moody and Emotional

When you're overly tired, do you tend to feel more overwhelmed, stressed, depressed, and downright cranky? If your answer is yes, you are not alone. New moms are at a higher risk of suffering from numerous mood and mental disorders, in addition to postpartum depression, related to extended sleep disturbances and exhaustion. A study published in *Journal of Obstetric, Gynecologic, & Neonatal Nursing* revealed that depression symptoms became exacerbated in postpartum women when there was a decline in their sleep quality and quantity.[8] The upside is that once you start getting enough quality sleep, your mood should return to normal. If not, be sure to discuss this with a trustworthy physician.

Research reveals that even small amounts of regular sleep deprivation can have a marked impact on our mood. One study performed by researchers at the University of Pennsylvania limited subjects to 4.5 hours of sleep each night. After just one week, subjects described themselves as feeling "more stressed, angry, sad, and mentally exhausted."[9] When getting back on normal sleep schedules, all subjects reported considerable improvements in their emotional stability and disposition.

The mood-sleep issue goes both ways. Your mental state and mood can also affect your sleep quality. When you are extra anxious or on edge (for example, constantly worried that your baby will die in his or her sleep, like I was with my first), your body will have a harder time relaxing and shutting down. Extended periods of stress, such as when you're caring for a colicky baby, can increase your brain stimulation, anxiety, and tension, also making it more difficult to sleep. Therefore, new moms need to look at this from two angles: We need to get more sleep so we can feel more happy and relaxed, and we need to feel more happy and relaxed so we can fall asleep. But how?

Here are a few tips that I have used successfully. Try them and see which ones work for you!

— *Do everything you can to get your baby on a good sleep schedule as soon as possible.* Some babies are great sleepers by nature, while others need guidance on how to sleep well. It is a huge benefit for both mother and baby when baby gets enough sleep. I've had one of each kind of sleeper. When I finally got serious about helping my first child sleep through the night, my entire outlook brightened greatly. She has become a fabulous sleeper overall, to this day.

— *Learn from great books on the subject of helping your children become good sleepers.* I found that *On Becoming Baby Wise: Giving Your Infant the Gift of Nighttime Sleep,* by Gary Ezzo and Robert Bucknam, presented a very simple concept that was most effective for good naps and the development of a routine. I used the method in *Solve Your Child's Sleep Problems,* by Dr. Richard Ferber, when my first child suddenly became a terrible sleeper at six months old. Within three (rough) nights, she became a fabulous sleeper and has been so ever since. *The No-Cry Sleep Solution: Gentle Ways to Help Your Baby Sleep Through the Night,* by Elizabeth Pantley, is an ideal book for parents who want a gentler alternative to the Ferber method.

— *Establish a bedtime routine for yourself, and do it earlier than normal.* Take a bath and have a cup of chamomile tea or wine. Turn off the TV and computer at least an hour before you go to bed. TVs, computer screens, and bright indoor lights emit blue light, just as the sun does. Our bodies, which can't tell the difference between natural and artificial light, limit the production of melatonin while exposed to blue light; therefore we stay wide awake and alert. This is a tough one for me. I used to spend time on the computer or watch *The Daily Show with Jon Stewart* with my hubby before bed. Now we view our favorite shows and use the computer a little earlier, and it feels like a better way to unwind. Basically, keep it mellow in the hours before bedtime.

— *Take time for quiet each day.* Whether you meditate for ten minutes or sit in the sun and close your eyes while you feed your baby, take time to simply be. This will help reduce anxiety—which will help you sleep better when you actually get the chance.

— *Sleep while the baby sleeps!* Everyone says this, but it is very wise advice and oh, so true. It is tempting to want to get some work done while the baby sleeps, and sometimes it is simply unavoidable. However, we need to make sure we are doing what we can to get at least 7 hours of sleep during every 24-hour period. If you have to, spend 30 minutes on housework or your favorite project and then curl up on the couch and grab a little shuteye. Or bring your laptop or project into bed and work until you feel sleepy; then simply drift off for some instant rejuvenation!

Nourishment: Key Two for Weight Loss Is Healthy Eating

Eating healthy foods is one of the most important things you can do to feel vibrant and full of energy. I urge you to think about treating your body as a maternal shrine! If you're nursing, you really need to think about the nutrition you're passing on to your baby. If you're not nursing, it is still crucial for you to eat well to continue to recover physically and to maintain your liveliness.

My best advice is to eat as naturally as possible. I like the ideas in Michael Pollan's *Food Rules: An Eater's Manual*. Some of Pollan's philosophies are similar to my own eating guidelines, which include the following:

- Eat food that's as close to its natural state as possible.

- Eat the freshest, most local food you can find.

- Eat as much organically grown food as you can (for health and environmental purposes). At a minimum, buy organic versions of the things you eat and drink the most, such as milk, bread, and certain fruits and vegetables. The Environmental Working Group (EWG) has published a list called the "Dirty Dozen" (**www .ewg.org/foodnews/summary/**), which might help you determine where to spend your money on organic produce.

- Minimize hard-and-fast rules other than to eat natural and whole foods as much as possible.

- Eat just enough to be satisfied.

- Eat a fruit and a vegetable at every meal.

- Don't deprive yourself of any favorite food; if it's not good for you, just make eating it more of a rare and special occasion.

In my opinion, dieting is a way of telling your subconscious that something is wrong with you. You are essentially depriving yourself by eliminating "bad" foods or counting every calorie. This isn't to say you should eat whatever you want; rather, I suggest you simply examine how you eat. Are you eating foods that benefit your body the majority of the time? If so, then I think you're doing great in this area. Eat until you are full, and then stop. Don't deprive yourself, because then you will just want the forbidden food even more.

If you don't eat too much and you eat healthfully but the scale is not budging toward your ideal weight, then maybe you need to reevaluate the other three pieces of the weight loss puzzle (sleeping, exercising, and body love). Since we are all doing this program to get our bodies back to their ideal weight and condition after giving birth, we have to simply try to do better.

I just cannot go on a diet. It's psychological. If I say, "I am on a diet," I start obsessing about food all day long. Conversely, if I say to myself, "I am going to eat well this week" or "I am going to eat more fruit this week and have wine only on the weekend," I do a much better job. It also really helps to have a lot of healthy and easy-to-prepare food on hand. When you are busy, stressed, and tired, you will stand looking in your cupboards, searching for the simplest and fastest food to give you satisfaction. If it's a Snickers bar or a bag of chips, that's what you will grab. If none of that is in your cupboard, you won't miss it—especially if you have healthy alternatives on hand, such as yummy hummus with carrots or a jar of sea-salted almonds.

In conclusion, love your body and stop filling it with processed, toxic foods that do not promote your vitality and well-being! Make junk food an occasional snack. It's funny: when I do eat junk now, after a brief high, I end up feeling crummy, and my energy plummets. Consider eating mostly foods that you'd want your children to eat.

Fitness: Key Three to Weight Loss Is Exercise

Exercising is imperative for losing your baby weight and getting your muscles toned and lean. We are going to start getting our bodies back in a nice and gentle way, with our focus on making the body feel limber and agile once again. Start to get in the habit of doing some form of exercise on most days. I recommend a lot of walking, gentle stretching, and yoga as you get started. Strength exercises can include any toning or strengthening moves that use your own body weight such as squats, pushups, and Pilates. You can accelerate your muscle building and toning by adding pounds to your strength exercises by using free weights, participating in weight-lifting classes, or using weight machines at the gym.

Be patient, and be kind to your body. Keep your expectations real, and honor that your body is still recuperating. Getting "ripped" should not be your first priority at this time; keeping healthy and promoting healing should be most important.

Please remember that the workout schedule for Week 1, below, is for women who have recovered completely from birth and are ready to start getting back into shape. Keep in mind that this exercise schedule is an ideal, and babies often make working out every day difficult to accomplish. I urge you to do what you can, and slowly work up to getting yourself into a regular exercise routine. Furthermore, this book is written in a weekly format for those who want to stick to a schedule, but you can use it at the speed that works best for you.

Exercising for mental clarity and sanity is often important for athletic mothers, but try to keep exertion light and comfortable at all times. There will be plenty of time in another month or so for high-impact exercise. For now, choose exercises that are gentle and that allow your joints, ligaments, and uterus to heal completely. Don't forget that your intelligent body has been producing the hormone relaxin, which had the great purpose of softening the cervix and increasing tissue and joint flexibility to help with the birthing process. This hormone lingers for quite some time after birth, which means you need to be particularly gentle with stretching, and later with more active weight-bearing exercise. Not only is your body in a major recovery process, but this hormone also renders it more susceptible to injury.

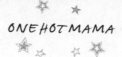
Week 1 Workout Schedule

Monday	Tuesday	Wednesday	Thursday	Friday	Saturday	Sunday
30-minute walk	15 minutes strength	45-minute walk or low-impact cardio class at gym	15 minutes strength	30-minute walk or low-impact cardio class at gym	Yoga or Pilates class	Rest

Gentle Yoga Workout

Yoga fits perfectly into the recovery process and can slowly ease you back into fitness. It also helps calm and clear your mind, which can be fuzzy from being so darn tired. Focusing on your breath while lightly stretching will help you feel better, sooner. Yoga is also important to really open up and stretch your chest, to compensate for all the hours you spend hunched over feeding and gazing down at your sweet baby. I remember after a few weeks of nursing, my neck was very sore from tilting to the left and looking down at the same time. I've heard other moms complain of headaches and knots in their necks and shoulders. A nice massage could certainly alleviate this pain, too! I could barely roll my neck around until I started doing yoga daily. Just do what feels good!

My top seven recommended postnatal poses are:

1. *Kegel Exercises.* Nora Isaacs, yoga instructor, mom, and former editor at *Yoga Journal*, recommends Kegel exercises to improve the strength of the pelvic floor, which can be weakened during pregnancy and childbirth. Isaacs says, "These contractions correct incontinence and strengthen the pelvic floor."[10] Kegel exercises aid the healing process by increasing blood flow to the uterus and associated organs without stress or pressure. *To do:* Pick your position: cross-legged, Child's Pose, or lying on your back. Then quickly squeeze the muscles that stop the flow of urine. Make the contractions progressively longer: Squeeze for a count of five, hold for five, and release for five. Repeat ten times.

2. *Wide-Legged Forward Bend (Prasarita Padottanasana).* This pose is amazing for releasing tension in the neck, shoulders, back, and hamstrings. I like to just relax in this posture, while enjoying the feeling of increased space between the vertebrae of my neck. This position is calming and is touted as being able to help remedy headaches and mild depression. *To do:* Set your feet about three to four feet apart, and place your hands on your hips. Make sure to keep your feet parallel while firmly pressing your big toes and the outer edges of your feet into the floor. Slowly lean forward from your hips while exhaling. You can grab your elbows and let the weight of your body pull you down, or you can rest your head and hands on the floor, letting your head pull naturally toward the ground. Stay in this pose for up to a minute before placing your hands on your hips and slowly returning to an upright position.

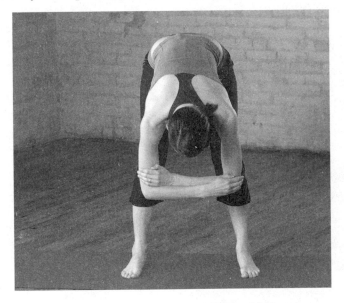

Wide-Legged Forward Bend, demonstrated by Laura,
hot mama of Benjamin and Alex

3. *Cat Pose and Cow Pose (Marjaryasana and Bitilasana).* I like using these two poses together to stretch my entire neck and upper back. These poses are also known for massaging internal organs and getting blood flowing to help heal your uterus. When done in conjunction with breathing, this is one of the most relaxing vinyasas (flows of yoga poses) that you can do. *To do:* Kneel on all fours, keeping your hands directly below your shoulders and your knees straight down from your hips at a 90-degree angle. Start with Cat Pose by dropping your head and rounding your spine toward the sky, creating a nice, deep stretch in your neck and back. Then gently move into Cow Pose as you inhale. To do Cow Pose, arch your back downward and stretch your rear end as high as you can while lifting your neck and chest up and looking toward the sky. Inhale deeply into this pose. Repeat this sequence with your breathing 20 times.

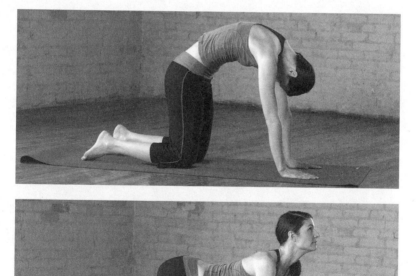

4. *Gentle Seated Twist (Bharadvajasana I).* This pose really focuses on stretching the hips, upper shoulders, neck, and lower spine. It also relieves stress and is known to help digestion. I use this pose to focus on stretching areas that are particularly tight from holding my baby or from using the computer too much. *To do:* Start this pose by sitting on the floor with your legs straight out in front of you. Shift your weight over to the right and bend your knees to bring your feet around to the left, so that you can place your heels close to your left buttock. Rest your left ankle in the arch of your right foot. As you inhale deeply, lift the top of your head toward the sky to lengthen your spine. As you exhale, twist your torso to the right while using your left arm to help twist your body on your right thigh near your knee. Place your right hand on the floor behind you near your buttock as you look in that direction. As you inhale, continue to lift through the top of your head, and then press further into the twist with every exhalation. Hold this position for about 30 seconds, release with an exhale, and switch sides.

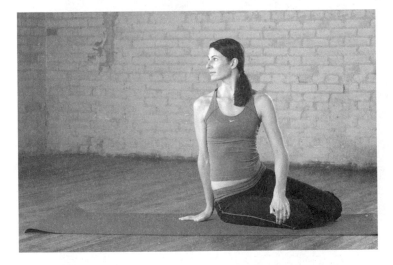

5. *Legs Up the Wall Pose (Viparita Karani). Yoga Journal* states that ancient and modern yoga teachers alike have believed that this pose can relieve just about everything, including tired or cramped legs and feet; headaches; and tension in the back of the legs, torso,

and back of the neck.[11] It also nicely calms the mind. It is just a wonderful way to relax, meditate, and let go of any tension! *To do:* This pose can be done with props such as a bolster under the small of your back or a lavender-scented eye pillow but is just as effective with nothing but a wall. Sit a few feet from the wall with your feet touching the bottom of the wall. "Walk" up the wall as you scoot your bottom to where the wall and floor meet. Your body should be in a 90-degree angle. Let your arms rest loosely out, with your palms facing up. The main effort will be keeping your legs straight up the wall; otherwise, just let your body relax and melt into the floor; let your eyes close and "look" toward your heart. Stay in the pose, breathing deeply for up to five minutes. When you come out of the pose, lie on one side for a few seconds before getting up very slowly.

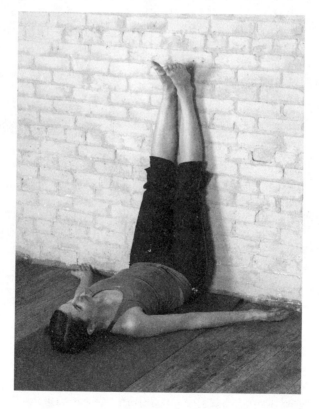

6. *Child's Pose (Balasana).* This relaxing pose is perfect for relieving back pain, stretching your hips, and releasing your shoulders. It's a great pose in which to sit and relax while focusing on your breath. *To do:* Kneel, sitting back on your heels, toes pointing back. Bend forward and place your forehead on the ground. Release all the tension in your neck, back, and torso, and let it sink down toward the ground. Position your arms along your body with your palms facing up, straight out on the floor above your head, or however feels comfortable to you. Sit as long as it feels good, and take deep breaths, visualizing oxygen filling up and healing the spaces where you are sore and tight. Slowly roll up.

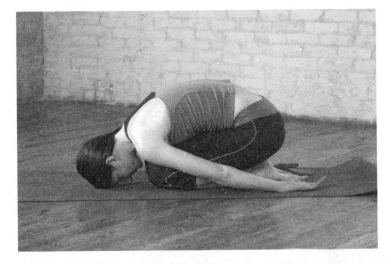

7. *Corpse Pose (Savasana).* Savasana is my favorite ending to any yoga class or practice. I savor it. And yes, it's as easy to do as it sounds. The goal is to relax each part of your body—every single muscle and your heart, brain, internal organs, eyeballs, jaw, tongue, and skin. I start by going through my entire body and searching for tension. Then I try to release it as much as possible. As your breathing slows and your body slips into relaxation, your mind will either race, wander, or fall into a deeply relaxed state. Just bring your mind back to your breath if it wanders. You may

want to focus on a word such as *love* or visualize something beautiful or calming to you. *To do:* Lie on your back, with your feet spaced comfortably apart and toes falling to the sides naturally. Let your hands fall to the sides, palms up. The goal is to get your body as comfortable and neutral as possible. I often like to put a blanket or pillow under my knees. Relax your entire body, and breathe naturally. Stay in this pose for about five minutes if you can. When you're ready to get up, roll to one side and stay curled up for a few seconds before pushing up to a seated position.

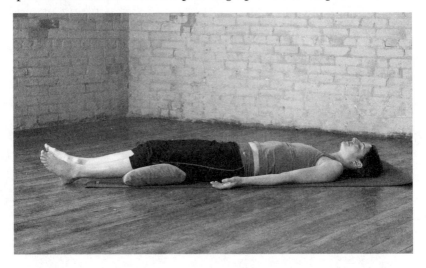

Appreciating Your Body: Key Four to Weight Loss Is Body Love

I believe that loving yourself and your body is such an important—and frequently overlooked—component of weight loss. When you look at your body with disgust and criticize various features, you are sending your subconscious mind a very powerful negative message. Your subconscious mind does not know or care whether these thoughts are true; it simply believes them. When you have convinced yourself that you are heavy and loathsome, then you will subconsciously self-sabotage to remain in that condition.

You cannot hate your body and treat it with love at the same time. I know many women whose mantra is, "I am fat, and no matter what I do, I seem to stay this way." Then, when they go on a diet or exercise, if they don't see results quickly enough, they go back to their bad habits right away. Therefore, they remain the same size, making their prediction come true.

I don't believe there are many women out there who adore their cellulite or back fat, but if you have a deep appreciation for your body overall and express self-love, you will set yourself up for real change. Don't focus on the cellulite if it bothers you. Focus on the facts—for example, that you rarely get sick, you have strong arms, and you are able to bear children. Then send your body gratitude for these things.

Visualization is a powerful tool for change. Love yourself so much that you can visualize yourself looking your most fit and energized. Then nourish your body with healthy food and exercise until your vision becomes reality. Picture yourself at your very best, and send positive and exciting thoughts toward looking that way again.

Sanity Saver: The Happiness Habit

Happiness is attainable for moms, of course, but in general, it requires more self-care, organization, and effort than before. While being a mom will bring you some of your highest highs, it might also bring you some of your lowest lows. It can introduce more work into your daily life as well as stress and strain into your marriage. Exhaustion also plays a huge factor in feeling unhappy and overwhelmed.

One of the biggest keys to happiness as a mom is living in the moment and being completely present with whomever you're with or the task at hand. This can be tough when your mind is racing about all of your unfinished tasks. When you find your thoughts running rampant, take a few deep breaths and bring yourself 100 percent back to the present moment. It is so beautiful and life changing when you figure out how to snap yourself into fully experiencing your life!

Sit down with a pen and paper and really figure out what brings you satisfaction and joy. Does your writing reveal that you miss time pursuing your passions or how much you love fashion, singing, dancing, or taking pictures? Is it most important for you to spend focused time with your children each day? Do you want to make your relationship with your husband a bigger priority in your life? Then try to live in a way that is in alignment with these things as much as possible.

Of course, a neat and clean house is important, but you cannot let yourself stress about it all day long—or sacrifice your happiness for it. Kids make houses messy, so you might as well wait until the end of the day to pick everything up. As your children grow up, be sure to train them to pick up after themselves.

I have a few tasks to do around the house every morning and evening, but in between I do not think about them. I used to find myself ruminating about the dirty dishes and laundry piling up all day long, when I should have been enjoying my kids. It's easy to let the myriad of household tasks overwhelm you to the point that you don't enjoy your relationships or what you are doing in the moment. My constant clean in the evening and feeling as though I couldn't relax until everything was perfect used to drive my husband crazy. He just wanted me to chill out with him at the end of a long day.

Every day is different, and sometimes you just have to let things go. As I write this paragraph, sitting at my kitchen barstool, I look around and see that I've really let things go this week to the point where it is starting to affect my happiness and sense of inner peace. The sink has a few dirty dishes, the floor beneath my preschooler's spot at the table is full of crumbs, and the counter has a pile of unread mail and my kindergartner's papers from her week at school. It has been a long week at work, and tonight I would love to sit here with my favorite dark chocolate and my new laptop, imagining and then writing about how I can contribute to making the world a better place. However, things in my house have gotten to the point where it is no longer peaceful. I am going to balance my time by listening to an awesome podcast for a half hour while getting my house under control. I will do as much as I can in that time, and then I will just have to live with the rest of the mess until tomorrow.

Another key to happiness is nurturing your interests and relationships outside of your children. My greatest hope is that I can inspire moms to take better care of themselves and maintain what makes them great as individuals, not just as good moms. Being yourself and staying fabulous and interesting only makes you a better mother. Being happy is contagious, and being joyful and present sets a great example for your children. How you treat yourself will teach your children how to treat themselves. Devoting yourself completely to your children while neglecting yourself will not benefit anyone in the long run. I am not saying that you should neglect your children but rather that you should care for and love yourself so you can better care for and love your family.

Plan things to look forward to each day, such as fun outings with your girlfriends and kids. Explore your surroundings to find the best places to take a newborn and your older kids, such as a local library or park. Meet a friend for coffee. Find joy in little rituals like sipping a delicious cup of tea or watering your beautiful flowers. Be present with your family, and don't get bogged down in the minutiae of everyday life. Get up and seize each day!

One thing that has brought me so much joy is praying or meditating early in the morning before my family wakes up. When the children get out of bed, our morning ritual is to snuggle up and read a few of their favorite books in my comfy chair by a big window. It starts the day out right, in contrast to the mornings where we all sleep in and have to rush somewhere.

In conclusion, here are a few tips for creating a happy life:

- Establish comforting rituals.

- Enjoy the little things, and be fully present in the moment.

- Organize your surroundings.

- Take good care of your health by eating well and getting as much rest and exercise as you can.

- Make time for fun outings with your kids and with other moms.

- Get a babysitter once in a while and go out with a girlfriend for a no-child lunch—then maybe a pedicure, if your budget allows.

- Meet a friend or your man at a coffee shop for some good conversation.

- Turn on your favorite music.

- Grab a glass of wine and a square of chocolate, and watch your favorite TV show.

- Sit down and give your children your full attention, and see how happy it makes them, which will make you feel happy, too.

- Go for a walk.

- Read a wonderful book with your baby snuggled next to you.

- Cuddle with your children in bed and read books to them.

- Call your best friend or mother.

Take the time to really enjoy your life as a mother. Strive to see your new child as a gift that brings you great joy and pushes you to grow as a woman. At the same time, acknowledge that being a mom is not the only thing that defines you. You are still the same talented, beautiful woman with something very special to offer the world. Don't forget that woman, and don't forget that you are *One Hot Mama*!

Affirmation for the Week

You may choose to read this affirmation out loud or to yourself, to reaffirm what you have learned this week.

As I go through the process of "getting myself back" after such a major life event, I vow to have patience, self-love, and compassion. I will practice looking at my body with appreciation and gratitude for all it has been through. I will take care of this beautiful woman and will stay motivated to stick with this process. I am worth it!

★☆★

Money Talks

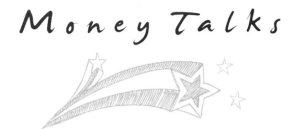

*"Money is only a tool. It will take you wherever you wish,
but it will not replace you as the driver."*

— AYN RAND

How many times do you use or think about money each day?
It takes money to put gas in your car, purchase groceries for your
family, and pay your mortgage or rent. Having enough money is
crucial for living and for raising children. Unfortunately, money is
often overlooked as an issue of importance for moms. In my own
experience as well as that of most women I know, a woman's earning potential is at a critical changing point after having children.

After having my first baby, I continued to work, but I used my
full maternity leave and 12 weeks of Family and Medical Leave Act
(FMLA) time—which meant my salary was cut more than in half
for that first year. This was quite an adjustment and made me realize how much I equated my success and power with the money I
earned. I am not a particularly materialistic person, but since I had
worked for nearly a decade before becoming a mom, I was used to
pulling my weight financially and being able to spend money how
I chose. Since having my children, I have never earned as much
as I did pre-baby. That's generally just fine with me, but it has certainly required significant lifestyle changes, ego adjustment, and
personal growth.

Debt and inadequate funds are particular concerns and sources of stress for many moms, whose main goal in life is to have
enough so their families live comfortably. In fact, depression and

debt are inextricably linked in mothers. Financial strain is also a real stressor in marriages and is often cited as one of the top five causes of divorce. We need to come to peace with money, and what we earn or don't earn, in order to live our most peaceful and joyful lives.

Your Relationship with Money

Before having children, I had always considered money only moderately important—something necessary to pay my bills and purchase the things I needed and wanted. What I have come to realize as an adult is that I have a strained relationship with money. Growing up, my parents did not include my brother or me in any money discussions, and I never stressed about the cost of anything. We were a middle-class family and certainly not rolling in dough, but my parents felt that money was something kids shouldn't think or worry about. It was wonderful to grow up sheltered, but as I grew older, it created some issues for me.

During graduate school, I lived in downtown Minneapolis on a modest graduate assistant stipend and finally learned by experience what it really took to live. After paying rent and bills, I had about $200 per month to live on. On some months I could make this work, but in others I would get caught up spending far too much in the spirit of the holiday season or have an unexpected expense (like fixing my roommate's car, which I hit while trying to parallel park). Then I would have to use my newly minted credit card for necessities, like groceries. I also got the idea to spend a month in Europe after graduate school because it might be the last big chunk of time I would have with no job or other major commitments in my life. I used a student loan to fund this once-in-a-lifetime trip.

What I didn't account for were the costs that would come after I returned from my European tour, including moving to California, furnishing an apartment, and purchasing professional clothes. My salary sounded great until I started living on exclusive

Balboa Island in a great little apartment a block from the water. Needless to say, I didn't have much money left over each month after paying off my student loan and credit card debt. My feelings about money included frustration, fear, and deprivation. I was discouraged because I felt like I could never get ahead. I started feeling guilty every time I made a purchase, no matter how much money was in my account.

Money is a form of energy. It is required to purchase everything we need to live. While many of us may not necessarily be materialistic, we want the comfortable lifestyle that money affords. If you have an unhealthy relationship with money, you must repair it in order to live your happiest life, particularly since money can become an emotional issue tied to self-worth if you are working less or taking time off to focus on being a mother.

Research has shown that money concerns and debt are strongly correlated with depression in mothers.[1] This result doesn't surprise me, because moms care more about providing for their family than just about anything else. If we feel insecure in our financial well-being and fear that we may not be able to provide necessities for our children, this constant psychological stress can lead to a depressed condition. Don't minimize the importance of your emotional connection to your finances.

I have been working on my relationship with money for many years now, with my husband. We do not have major money concerns, but we can't spend like crazy or have the lifestyle we dream of quite yet. We feel thankful that we are able to save some and give some. Developing a detailed budget so I know exactly how much I can spend on things has made life so much better for me, but I am still working to minimize the feelings of lack and guilt that have plagued me since my post–graduate school days.

In order to have a peaceful and friendly relationship with money, we need to put a lot of positive energy toward judicious spending and saving. Now that I have a budget, I can either spend a little each month or save up for a few months to splurge on a larger item! It is incredibly empowering to be in control of money, and I wish I had had the discipline to accomplish this years ago. It feels very powerless not to have any control over your spending. If that's how you feel, sit down with your partner and say you want to be equally involved in your family's finances.

First, you have to work to eliminate unnecessary debt. Unfortunately, "fun" spending needs to be limited until the debt is gone. Debt can leave people feeling stressed and depressed, and is a major source of marital discontent. A lot of the guilt I felt about money occurred when I would buy something that didn't feel completely necessary, like new clothes, while knowing I owed money on a credit card. That kind of spending didn't feel authentic or right in my soul. Developing healthy spending and saving habits is the first step toward having a powerful relationship with money. Only after you have a good plan to take care of your debt can you move toward being generous with your money—using it to help others or to enrich your lifestyle.

Putting positive thoughts and energy toward the things you'd like to have will honestly help those things come your way. My husband is a master at fixating on one thing at a time until it materializes in his life. This technique has worked for him in so many ways, from getting to fly his dream plane at work every day to purchasing the latest and greatest HD video camera. He researches and concentrates on one thing with laser focus until it is his.

I am starting to do this, too, and I find that it helps me focus my spending on what I really want. For a while, all I really desired was a comfortable and beautiful home. I looked around and realized that I had a beautiful house; it just needed a few decorating touches. I saved up money and spent it on an interior decorator, who gave me advice on a few small things I could do to make the house look more polished. Now the place feels so much better to me. Next I am going to focus on my workout clothes. I will find exactly the pieces I want and determine the cost; then I will save accordingly. I have been doing this with all the things I want, from beauty products to jogging strollers. I find that I am so much more satisfied with my purchases because they are things I really desire, and I do my homework before buying them.

Here are a few useful tips that have worked well for me and may help you improve your relationship with money:

— Remember that money has the power to bring you the lifestyle you desire.

— Debt needs to be managed before it leads to feelings of helplessness, depression, and marital issues.

— Budgets can help you feel empowered so you know how much you can spend each month and still meet your family's financial goals.

— Make sure your spending is in alignment with your morals and goals in life. You should be spending your money on what's most important to you.

— If you're not in a position to spend a lot of money right now, relax because there are so many ways to live well on a budget. (Think consignment stores, libraries, movie nights at home, and living simply.)

— Be happy with and proud of who you are. Forget about the pressure to "keep up with the Joneses." Anyone who thinks that possessing a nicer, newer car (or fill in the blank) makes them better than you is someone you do not need in your life.

Nourishment: Eating Well While Eating Out!

Eating at restaurants or ordering takeout food once in a while is fun and convenient. We can all occasionally use a night off from cooking dinner, and going out to nice restaurants on dates or with girlfriends is simply a pleasurable part of life. I discuss this at length in Week 3's section on social eating, but eating out can be more complicated and cause setbacks when trying to lose weight.

Therefore, I want to offer a few useful tips and pose a few questions for you to keep in mind here.

Select restaurants that you know have some good options. When you go out, I am guessing you have at least a few choices to select from. I live in a smaller town, and we still have numerous restaurants. A few places literally do not have one healthy thing on the menu—only fried food and iceberg/cheese/ranch types of salads. While they have good beer, I know when I go there that I will not be eating anything nourishing. I try not to eat real meals there or go there hungry. On the other hand, there are places with some grilled, broiled, and fresh options. There are dishes that will taste absolutely delicious that aren't fried and don't have heavy sauces. A menu will always offer some items that are better for you than others; the key is to order the better meals.

Take your time while looking at the menu. Don't rush and order impulsively. Take your time and pick something that both sounds good and will be somewhat healthy and nourishing.

Practice portion control. This is so cliché, but I will say it again. Don't eat too much! In general, restaurants serve twice as much as the average woman probably needs to eat. I am a cardholder in the clean-plate club, but I am not as proud of that fact now that I don't weigh 120 pounds. It has taken a lot of effort and practice not to blindly clean my plate. Look at your food and imagine how much you should eat before you dig in. Eat slowly, and give your body time to notice whether it has had enough. Share meals, or take some home for a yummy lunch tomorrow. Or eat it all now but then eat smaller meals for the rest of the day.

Think about how you will feel after you eat. I started doing this during pregnancy, when eating the wrong thing would make me feel absolutely terrible for a few hours afterward. I discovered that eating processed and super-greasy food tasted pretty good, but I'd end up with wicked heartburn and indigestion. As I get older, I find that I feel lethargic, bloated, and crappy overall after an especially fatty meal.

When you start eating bad food, you will crave it more. Over lunch the other day, one of my best friends told me all about her vacation to Costa Rica. She described the amazing hiking, kayaking, and other adventures, but one thing that stood out to her was how energized and vibrant she felt while there. She ate only meals of rice and beans with vegetables and fruit. At first she said she craved sugar and missed dessert. As a physical therapist, she has sweet treats every afternoon to keep her energy up during her 12-hour shifts. After a few days, she realized she no longer cared about sugar and felt absolutely amazing. She returned home to the United States shortly before the holidays and quickly fell back into eating sugar. However, she realized that she was better off without it, and after the holidays, she worked to cut it out of her diet again. The point is, the more sugar and fat you eat, the more your body craves them. When you cut them out of your diet, after a few days of cravings, you will realize your energy levels are more consistent and you simply feel better overall.

Fitness: Essential Gear and Getting Out There

There are two critical things for new mothers to have to facilitate regular workouts: great sports bras and smooth strollers. Since your chest is likely a little larger than usual, and potentially a lot more sensitive, it is crucial to have your breasts bound pretty securely to enjoy exercising.

Bracing the Breasts

There are two really important reasons to wear good bras: your comfort and preventing saggy boobs. Nursing is hard enough on the chest, so we need to be extra careful to protect our breasts during bouncy exercise. Research has shown that an unsupported A-cup breast will bounce an inch and a half in every direction, while D cups can travel two to three inches every which way. Wow! Good bras are shown to cut bouncing in half, so before picking up the walking pace and especially before you start jogging, invest in a few new bras to protect your chest and keep the girls perky.

I will share what to look for in a good sports bra. While your breasts are larger, I recommend an encapsulation-type of sports bra. It sounds scary, I know, but it will keep the girls in place better than any other. Racerback bras keep the breasts closer to the body, but wider, straight straps might be better while your breasts are larger because they distribute the weight better. I also recommend finding a bra that has a back clasp, which will provide a little extra support.

It is also crucial to get the best size for you. After having my first child, I crammed my two-sizes-bigger breasts into my regular sports bras and just put on two of them. This can work okay, although it can be hard to breathe! Once I purchased some pricier, high-quality bras and felt the difference, I couldn't go back.

My personal favorite sports bra is Moving Comfort (Maia High Impact, with a back closure). The company's website even has a cool tool to help you select the right bra for you based on your size and the sports you will be doing.

One of Your Best Investments: A Good Jogging Stroller

I have tried numerous strollers, and there is a massive difference between the low- and high-end ones. When I was a mother of one, I used a phil&teds, and it worked fairly well for running. It had a jump seat for the older child when another baby came along, but then I could not run with it very well. When my second child arrived, I did a lot of research and surveyed dozens of friends, and I ended up with the BOB Revolution Duallie. They are not cheap and are difficult to find used. However, I use the darn thing so much that it has been one of the best baby investments my husband and I have made. You can run with two children very smoothly, and the shock system and handling are phenomenal.

I recommend that you do a lot of research using books, consumer websites, and mommy blogs, as well as by asking your friends. Then buy the very best stroller you can afford. Try out your girlfriends' strollers to see which one feels smooth and right for you. A great stroller will motivate you to get outside and use it!

Picking Up the Pace

Last week, we started slow with some gentle yoga and stretching. This week, we are going to start picking up the pace. Please tailor the actual exercises to your current fitness level. The main goal this week is to increase the frequency and duration of your workouts.

Aim to do a minimum of four workouts this week, but strive for five or even six (as shown in the Week 2 Workout Schedule, below) if you can manage it. Select workouts that fit your schedule, preferably two strength workouts and two or more cardio workouts. Here are some suggestions:

- Cardio workouts include walking, jogging, running, biking, low-impact aerobics, dancing, and hiking.

- Strength workouts include Pilates, yoga, free weights, stroller strength workout, and weight classes (using light weights).

Do the best you can. This is an idealistic starting point from which to set your exercise goals. I know it's tough when you're sleep deprived and potentially feeling overtasked, but I promise that you will feel better after your workouts than you did before.

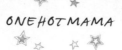
Week 2 Workout Schedule

Monday	Tuesday	Wednesday	Thursday	Friday	Saturday	Sunday
30-minute walk	15 minutes strength	45-minute walk or low-impact cardio class at gym	15 minutes strength	30-minute walk or low-impact cardio class at gym	Yoga or Pilates class	Rest

Stroller Strength-Building Workout

First, be sure to warm up with either a nice walk or a quick jog. This workout can also be done after a longer cardio workout if you've got the energy. Do this workout routine two or three times through, and finish up with a five-minute stretch.

1. *Walking Lunges.* With your hands lightly holding on to your stroller, lunge forward with alternating legs, making sure your back is straight, head is held high, and knees do not go past your toes. Put a majority of your weight on your heels, and really squeeze your rear as you straighten up. Do 20 lunges on each leg.

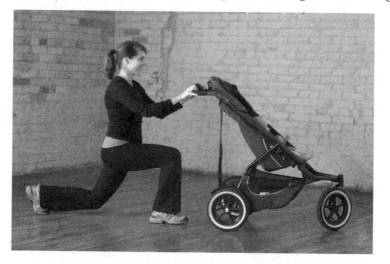

Walking Lunges, shown by Leah, hot mama of Greta
(our three-month-old model) and Ike

2. *Squats.* Stand with your feet about hip-width apart and your hands lightly holding on to your stroller. Squat down until your thighs are parallel with the ground, pushing your rear back as far as you can. The stroller will rock back and forth as you move up and down. Do 20 squats.

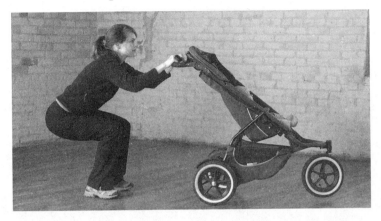

3. *Kick Backs Behind the Stroller.* For the next two exercises, think of yourself as a ballerina and your stroller as the barre. Put the brake on your stroller, and hold on lightly with both hands as you lift your right leg up to a 90-degree angle, with the gluteal and quadriceps flexed and your knee facing slightly outward. Repeat 20 times on each leg.

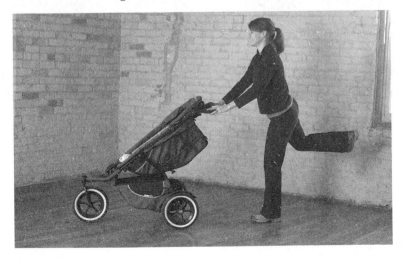

4. *Plié Squats.* Start with your feet about three feet apart and your knees facing out. Holding lightly on to your stroller with both hands, plié down until your thighs are parallel to the floor and your quadriceps are fully engaged. Hold for a breath, and use your muscles to straighten up slowly. Repeat 25 times. To mix it up, try alternating going up on your toes while doing the pliés.

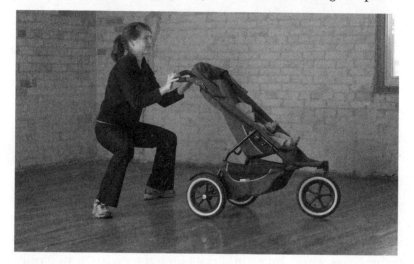

5. *Side Stroller Push-Pull.* Begin by standing perpendicular to your stroller with your right hand holding on to the handle. Stand with your feet a little more than hip-width apart. Take the brake off, and reach overhead as far as you can with your left arm, stretching through the entire left side of your torso. You will pull the stroller slightly toward you with your right arm as you stretch overhead further toward the stroller. Hold for a breath when you are stretching as far as you can, and then use your muscles to pull

the left arm all the way back so that your left elbow stretches to your left hip. You will be pushing the stroller away with your right arm as you come down. Repeat 25 times on each side.

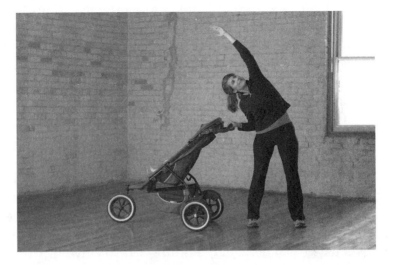

Sanity Saver: Journaling

I highly recommend purchasing a beautiful journal that you can use to record little bits of your new life as a mom. I went to a bookstore and bought a beautiful book that says, "Yesterday is history, tomorrow is a mystery, today is a gift." I love this saying from Eleanor Roosevelt, and writing in the book reminds me regularly to stay in the moment and be completely present for my children. I recommend that you keep a journal by your bed so you can scribble little items here and there before you pass out at night. You will be much more likely to capture the sweet daily memories this way than if you wait to write them all in a baby book.

I started jotting down little things, such as how my daughter's first smile amazed me and melted my heart and how watching my husband play with our daughter filled me with deep joy and satisfaction. I also described milestones for both me and my baby. I remember writing about the first time I got both of us up, dressed, and out of the house by 9 A.M. for a doctor's appointment. It was a big deal to me at the time and something I may have just forgotten otherwise. Take a few minutes as often as you can to capture the seemingly small things that will be precious to you one day.

Journaling is also a good way to check in with yourself to see how you're really doing—and to release emotions, if necessary. There were times (and still are) when I was really frustrated, feeling like I did everything in my house. My husband is an Air Force fighter pilot, and his incredibly busy and generally inflexible work schedule left me alone a lot to deal with all the parenting, cooking, cleaning, and shopping—in addition to trying to work a few hours a day. I had absolutely nothing left for myself. I felt unbalanced, like an emotional wreck. I knew my husband couldn't control his work schedule, but I was harboring resentment toward him nonetheless. One evening I sat down and wrote in my journal furiously, as though a valve had been opened and pressure was being released. I felt so much better afterward and actually recognized that I was doing far too much and that something needed to give. I also realized that I was having a lot of anxiety about the prospect of going back to work at that time.

Sitting down and writing can really help you understand some of your underlying pressures, anxieties, and frustrations. Recognizing these issues is only half the battle. The next step is figuring out how to improve the situation, if possible—or at least how to cope with things better.

Scientific evidence shows that writing in a journal provides numerous benefits. Studies performed at the University of Texas have demonstrated that regular journaling boosts the immune system by strengthening T cells (T lymphocytes), which play several roles in protecting our immunity to illness and disease.[2]

Writing in a journal can open up your soul by connecting the two hemispheres of your brain. The act of writing accesses your left brain, which is analytical and rational.[3] While your left brain is occupied, your right brain is free to create, intuit, and feel. In sum, writing removes mental blocks and allows you to "use all of your brainpower to better understand yourself, others, and the world around you."[4] I think that is a beautiful way to sum up how starting a journal might help you find harmony during the beautiful but trying times of motherhood. In her article "The Health Benefits of Journaling," Maud Purcell described the following benefits of regularly writing in a journal:[5]

— *Use writing as a way to become clear on your thoughts and feelings.* Do you ever seem all jumbled up inside, unsure of what you want or feel? Taking a few minutes to jot down your thoughts and emotions (no editing!) will quickly get you in touch with your internal world.

— *Frequent writing helps you get to know yourself.* By writing regularly, you will get to know what makes you feel happy and confident. You will also become clear about situations and people who are toxic to you, which is important information for your emotional well-being.

— *Writing helps you deal with stress more effectively.* Writing about anger, sadness, and other painful emotions helps to release the intensity of these feelings. Then you will feel calmer and better able to stay in the present.

— *Writing helps you more effectively solve problems.* Typically, we problem-solve from a left-brained, analytical perspective. But sometimes the answer to a problem can only be found by engaging right-brained creativity and intuition. Writing unlocks these other capabilities and affords access to unexpected solutions to seemingly unsolvable problems.

— *Writing helps you resolve difficult situations with other people.* Writing about misunderstandings rather than stewing over them will help you understand another's point of view. And in doing so, you just may come up with a reasonable resolution to the conflict.

There are other types of journaling that can be as quick or as time intensive as you desire. I read a profound book called *Simple Abundance*, which suggests writing daily in a gratitude journal. The author, Sarah Ban Breathnach, proposes that you write down five things you're thankful for every day. I believe everyone can find a few minutes for such an exercise! It is a beautiful concept and will help you recognize just how blessed you really are. Some days this will be so easy, when things are going smoothly. Other days, when the baby's screaming, the bank account is getting low, bills are piling up, or you are in pain, this can be tough. On these days, you must find joy and beauty in very small and simple things.

You can always identify something to be grateful for, such as the flowers your neighbor brought, the frozen lasagna in your freezer, the gorgeous sunrise you were up to see, the smoothness of your baby's skin, the comfort of the hot water during a shower, the joke that made you giggle, the gifts for your baby you are now able to use, the fact that clean and safe water comes out of your faucets, and living in a place that is safe and free. There is always a multitude of things to be grateful for if you live in awareness of all the beauty that surrounds you.

I remember a day during the first month of being a mother when I was painfully exhausted and still sorer than I thought I should be after three weeks. My nipples were bleeding, my daughter had spit up blood (from the blood tainting my milk), and my husband was working another 12-hour day. I was very lonely, and I thought, *What am I possibly going to be thankful for today?* Then it came to me, as though God were speaking through the voice in my mind: I have an amazing family, including a mother who called to check on me this morning; I have a loving husband, who is working hard to support our family; I have a gorgeous and healthy baby; I have a warm, comfortable house with plenty of food; and I have safe water to drink. There they were—five perfectly good things to praise God for! This exercise made me a more grateful and respectful person, one who is able to find happiness despite the circumstances. What a gift that is!

Affirmation for the Week

I believe that I have abundance in my life despite possible changes in my earning potential or employment status. I may have fewer material gifts at this moment, but the authentic richness of my life has just increased in a way that is immeasurable.

★❑★

No Comparison!

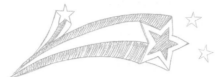

"You will make a lousy anybody else,
but you will be the best 'you' in existence."

— ZIG ZIGLAR

My mother: "I remember wearing my jeans home from the hospital after having you." Me: "Geez, how much weight did you gain?" Mom: "I gained about 19 pounds, but that's because I watched my weight and my doctor didn't want me to gain more than 20." Granted, this was in 1976 when doctors told women to diet while pregnant, while nowadays, doctors know better and recommend that healthy, average-sized women gain between 25 and 35 pounds during pregnancy.[1]

When my mom told me this story, I was about six months pregnant and had already gained 25 pounds! I felt like a big cow. I know Mom's account wasn't meant to make me feel bad, but it did. I thought of it many times over the year of being pregnant and getting back to normal again. When I returned home from the hospital after giving birth my first child, having gained somewhere between 35 and 40 pounds, I was still wearing a maternity sweat suit. There was no way I could have even gotten my regular jeans up my thighs! I finally relented and purchased larger clothes, releasing the unrealistic vision of going right back to my athletic fighting weight. But by the third month postpartum, I was feeling more like myself and could see the real potential for getting my body back to normal.

Body Image Is Rarely Challenged More Than After Having a Baby

Sadly, the way a woman feels about her appearance can have an incredible impact on her self-esteem and sense of self-worth. We will discuss spirituality and inner peace in later weeks, but now is the time to get you feeling really good about yourself. Feeling thin enough to wear your regular jeans and then pulling them on, only to find you can't quite get them buttoned, can be so defeating. Patience is hard to practice; however, it's the only way to maintain self-love and compassion until things return to normal.

It's easy to walk by the mirror and look at your body with disgust, feeling critical and wondering why the weight isn't coming off more quickly. During these moments, I urge you to think about the amazing feat your body has recently accomplished. Know that it took nine months to gain the weight required to nurture your baby to life, and for most women, it takes a good nine months or more to lose all the weight and get a tight and toned body. And that's if you're working at it.

Every time I am at the grocery store checkout, I see a magazine featuring a movie star posing in a bikini, looking better than ever only three months postpartum. These images can be defeating to many of us, causing us to wonder why we aren't looking anywhere near that fit that quickly. We could turn things around and see the images as motivational, giving those new moms kudos for working hard to look so good. Imagine how little they must have eaten and how hard they must have worked out. Also, please remind yourself that it's their job to be beautiful, and they have an entire cast and crew supporting them: trainers, dieticians, nannies, and stylists, to name just a few individuals. I am also guessing that many of those women are not nursing and are therefore able to cut calories to the point of being super hungry.

I personally couldn't cut back on calories significantly while nursing; otherwise, my milk production started dropping off. The same went for training really hard. I am a runner, and after my first baby was born, I started training for a half marathon when she was only three months old. After a week, I started realizing that she was continuously hungry and fussy—and I was exhausted and could hardly drag myself off the couch. So I cut back to training for a 10K and revamped my diet to make sure I was getting enough calories for both her and me. It was still really tough! When your baby is eating more solid food and is hopefully sleeping through the night, you can really pick up the intensity of your workout and start to feel more amazing each day.

Some women may tell you your body will never be the same again, but I see too many women who look even better after having children to believe it. The truth is, getting a tight, toned physique after giving birth requires effort . . . a lot of effort. You can lose all of the baby weight, but without yoga or toning exercises, a large majority of women will retain a flabby, loose stomach.

Women compare themselves to other women on a wide range of issues in addition to weight loss and body image, such as perceived parenting skills, clothing, job, and income (or lack thereof).

Sitting with any group of new mothers, you will hear one woman speaking with pride about the 50 bags of frozen breast milk she's got in her freezer because she produces so much she doesn't know what to do with it all! In the same room, there is a woman feeling inferior because her milk production is barely adequate and she is constantly concerned her baby isn't gaining weight quickly enough. One woman offers advice to the others because she's got her baby boy on a perfect schedule, sleeping 12 hours a night plus three long naps during the day. She offers her friends all kinds of unsolicited advice on how they can do things differently so their babies sleep better.

While it is often well intentioned, offering advice to other mothers on how they can do things better may cause them to feel insecure. Here is an example from my own experience. My baby was sleeping through the night by the age of seven weeks. Secretly feeling smug, I recommended the book *On Becoming Baby Wise,* by Gary Ezzo, to everyone; I honestly believed it could help all new mothers as much as it had helped me. Then all of a sudden, at six months, my baby started waking up three times a night, and there seemed to be nothing I could do to fix it. That quieted me in a hurry.

Many women feel insecure when they don't have a career to build their identity around, and they start feeling inferior to their moneymaking friends. My friend Marie complained recently to me that she wished there was some type of part-time job she could do from home to stimulate her mind and add to her family's bankroll. Many of her best friends have part-time jobs that are flexible and allow them to have what she perceives to be an ideal work-life balance. Marie finished graduate school right before giving birth to her first child, and she doesn't have any real work experience to get her foot in the door. I do know this: Staying home is an honorable and wonderful thing to do for your children. Marie is now trying to enjoy every moment with her children while taking small steps to keep her intellect challenged and dreaming about what she will do when she has more time as her children grow up.

If you are financially able to swing the arrangement of staying home to raise your children, try to consider it a blessing. If you are unsatisfied with your life, start brainstorming and journaling to become clear about what it is missing. Staying at home has its own benefits and drawbacks, as does working in any capacity. The key is to walk your own path, choose happiness where you are, and not compare yourself to your friends.

Focusing on Your Own Journey

I urge you to practice compassion and love toward your body. Regularly repeat the affirmation, "My body is strong, beautiful, and fit." Then take care of your health, exercise, and eat well until this statement becomes your reality. When you find yourself comparing your body and your weight loss journey to those of others, please stop and make a conscious effort to change your thoughts. I want you to focus only on yourself. You are in your own game, with your own unique body. As hard as it may be, I want you to make a deliberate effort to stop comparing yourself to anyone else.

I remember seeing a TV interview with Kate Hudson after she had her first child. Her story had a strong impact on me. Hudson had gained 60 pounds during her pregnancy. She said she was proud of it and that gaining weight to have a baby is "nothing to be ashamed of." Afterward, she didn't just shrink down magically; she actually had to work her tail off. She had to start filming a movie within three months of having her son, so she exercised two to three hours a day, running and working out with a trainer to lose the weight in time.

My friends, you, too, could lose weight that quickly if you had the time, help, and inclination to run on a treadmill for two to three hours a day. Kate Hudson said she would cry on the treadmill because of the pressure and the exhaustion she felt. I do not envy that kind of pressure, and I am thankful to have the luxury of losing baby weight in a way that is healthy, realistic, and sustainable.

Many Hollywood moms have to work incredibly hard to look as good as they do so quickly, but they want to make the transformation appear effortless in order to maintain their images. The problem is that this example can leave women of average means and metabolism feeling like failures. Do your best to stay in your own game and not compare your body or weight loss progress to those of anyone else.

The Pace of Your Weight Loss Journey

You will lose all the baby weight, and then some, if you are determined to do so. Have confidence in yourself, and find ways to continually motivate yourself to keep moving. We have unique bodies with individual metabolisms, emotional makeups, and weight loss challenges. The rate at which we get our bodies back to normal can vary dramatically from woman to woman. Keep in mind that there are many factors to consider, all of which have a major influence on your weight loss journey.

Metabolism

Does it ever feel like even if you eat less and exercise more than some of your friends, you still weigh more? There are so many things that affect your metabolism, or the rate at which your body burns calories, including genetics, diet, weight, and your muscle mass-to-fat ratio. There are clearly some items on this list that you cannot control; however, you can control what you eat, and you can start building muscle to increase the rate at which your body burns calories.

Body Type

Each of us is born with a beautiful and unique body type, and our goal should be to get as fit and slim as we can for our build. Some contend that women's bodies can never get back to being "perfect" after having a baby. The jury is still out on that one for me, but my body was never perfect before baby, so why would I have that unrealistic expectation afterward? There is certainly a part of me that would love to get back my high school body (I was a gymnast and track athlete), but I know the effort would be immense and I would have to do some serious dieting and intense exercising. Considering that I can barely fit in an hour for working out on most days, I am not sure this in the cards for me; but I will continue to try. I do believe that with enough effort and exertion, we can get our bodies back to what they were before baby—or even better if we're willing to put in the time and sweat.

Age

My sister-in-law has a younger sister who had her first baby in her early 20s, not long after I had my first child at 30. Within three months of delivering her daughter, she had posted tropical vacation photos of herself, looking toned and amazing in a bikini. My daughter was a few months older, I was nowhere near bikini ready, and the thought of anyone posting a photo of me in a bikini made me shudder! Your weight loss is affected not only by genetics and metabolism but also by age. As we age, our muscle density tends to decrease, which slows down the rate that our bodies burn calories. Did I mention that my mom, who wore her regular jeans home from the hospital when she had me, was only 20 at the time? I had my first child at 30, my second at 33, and my third at 35, and losing the weight seems to take slightly longer each time.

Identifying Your Weight Loss Challenge Areas

As I've been discussing, each of us is an individual, with unique a body type and challenges for weight loss. Take a few minutes to sit down and complete the following 25-question quiz. The results of this quiz will help you identify your weight loss challenge areas: unhealthy habits, emotional eating, social eating, mindless eating, lack of motivation to exercise, or a combination. The quiz will help you understand what factors might make it more difficult for you to lose weight. Then I will offer specific tips and tools to overcome your individual challenges.

Rate each of the following statements on a scale of 1 to 5, with 1 meaning you hardly relate and 5 meaning it sounds just like you!

UNHEALTHY HABITS

1. I have a shelf or drawer full of candy so I can have easy access to my favorite treats.

1 ☐   2 ☐   3 ☐   4 ☐   5 ☐

2. I have had the same eating habits since I was a child, and these are not the healthiest habits.

1 ☐   2 ☐   3 ☐   4 ☐   5 ☐

3. I eat sugary cereal or a granola bar on the go, or I often skip breakfast altogether.

1 ☐ 2 ☐ 3 ☐ 4 ☐ 5 ☐

4. I spend most of my time in the middle of the grocery store selecting easy-to-prepare processed, canned, and boxed food (as opposed to the fresh food around the edges).

1 ☐ 2 ☐ 3 ☐ 4 ☐ 5 ☐

5. I drink a lot of soda or other sugary drinks daily.

1 ☐ 2 ☐ 3 ☐ 4 ☐ 5 ☐

SCORE: _____

EMOTIONAL EATING

6. At the end of a long day, I want to curl up with a bag of chips or chocolate to relieve stress.

1 ☐ 2 ☐ 3 ☐ 4 ☐ 5 ☐

7. When I am under pressure and am feeling anxious, I crave my favorite comfort foods to make myself feel better.

1 ☐ 2 ☐ 3 ☐ 4 ☐ 5 ☐

8. I find myself eating much more comfort food than normal when I am fighting with my husband.

1☐ 2☐ 3☐ 4☐ 5☐

9. When I have been up all night with one of my children and am exhausted the next day, I seek food to give me a boost of energy.

1☐ 2☐ 3☐ 4☐ 5☐

10. During deadlines and times of duress, I increase my sugar and/or caffeine intake dramatically.

1☐ 2☐ 3☐ 4☐ 5☐

SCORE: _____

SOCIAL EATING

11. When I am invited to a friend's house for dinner, I clean my plate to make my host feel happy and show her my gratitude.

1☐ 2☐ 3☐ 4☐ 5☐

12. I go to parties and end up eating several plates of appetizers without thinking because I am caught up in good conversation and the jovial atmosphere.

1☐ 2☐ 3☐ 4☐ 5☐

13. When I am out with friends, I often unconsciously order foods similar to what everyone else is eating, even if the items are unhealthy and I would never order them on my own.

1 □ 2 □ 3 □ 4 □ 5 □

14. I would never speak up to convey specific dietary needs as a guest in someone's home or at a restaurant with friends.

1 □ 2 □ 3 □ 4 □ 5 □

15. When I am trying to watch what I eat, I sometimes find myself ordering something high in calories to fit in with what my dinner date is eating. I don't want to appear "not fun" by eating only a salad or a light meal.

1 □ 2 □ 3 □ 4 □ 5 □

SCORE: _____

MINDLESS EATING

16. I go to the grocery store when I'm hungry and end up buying way too much, often including unhealthy foods that I crave.

1 □ 2 □ 3 □ 4 □ 5 □

17. I sit down with a bag of chips to watch my favorite TV show, and before I know it, the bag is empty.

1 □ 2 □ 3 □ 4 □ 5 □

18. I often eat meals while deep in thought, not really paying attention or present. I end up eating way too much and not even enjoying the food because I am not really "there."

1☐ 2☐ 3☐ 4☐ 5☐

19. I often order the first thing that looks good on the menu, because I haven't really thought about it ahead of time. For example, at a coffee shop I see a chocolate croissant that looks delicious, so I order it impulsively.

1☐ 2☐ 3☐ 4☐ 5☐

20. I eat the same thing for breakfast every day, not because it's the healthiest meal or makes me feel amazing, but because I don't really think about it.

1☐ 2☐ 3☐ 4☐ 5☐

SCORE: _____

LACK OF MOTIVATION TO EXERCISE 21. I plan to exercise on many days but get too busy and just can't fit it in.

1☐ 2☐ 3☐ 4☐ 5☐

22. If I don't exercise first thing in the morning, I often feel too exhausted to do it as I get to the end of a long day.

1☐ 2☐ 3☐ 4☐ 5☐

23. I often make excuses, which may be legitimate in my mind, as to why I can't make it to the gym.

1 ☐ 2 ☐ 3 ☐ 4 ☐ 5 ☐

24. I've never belonged to a gym or haven't belonged to one in a really long time, and the thought of it intimidates me.

1 ☐ 2 ☐ 3 ☐ 4 ☐ 5 ☐

25. I'd like to exercise and know it would make me feel wonderful, but I am just not in the habit and have too many other things on my plate.

1 ☐ 2 ☐ 3 ☐ 4 ☐ 5 ☐

SCORE: _____

QUIZ RESULTS

If you scored over 15 in any of the weight loss challenge areas in the quiz, focus your attention on the associated solution section(s) below. It is good to be aware of your challenge areas so you can make conscious choices when faced with situations that make it difficult for you to eat well and exercise.

Solutions for Unhealthy Habits

Bad habits are really tough to break. When I was pregnant with my first child, I got in the habit of eating a bowl of ice cream or an ice cream sandwich every night. It became a comfortable ritual that I savored with my six-foot-five, thin, athletic husband, who can eat pretty much anything and not gain a pound. After the baby arrived, the ice cream habit was really tough to break because it had comforted me and I had thoroughly enjoyed it. It was especially difficult when my husband was able to continue eating ice cream every night, while for me it became an occasional treat.

Habits are formed because an act fulfills a perceived need. So if your habit is eating unhealthy junk food, try to figure out what's behind it. Do you feel lonely, bored, or scared? Are you seeking comfort? Are you subconsciously pursuing a boost in energy or happiness from food? Our food choices are often deeply rooted and are closely tied to our emotions.

If you have developed unhealthy habits over the span of a lifetime, it will take some time and effort to retrain your mind and your actions. It might be difficult, but the payoff is that you will feel more vibrant and energetic, and you will potentially lose weight.

Experts claim that it takes four to six weeks to make and break habits. Therefore, you will need to exert a conscious effort for over a month to make positive, long-term changes to what you put in your mouth. Here are a few tips to guide you through the process:

— *Replace the bad habit with a satisfying, healthy new habit.* For example, if your habit was eating a bag of Doritos every week while you watched *The Real Housewives of Orange County*, try eating a premeasured amount of sweet potato chips and put the rest of the bag away. Enjoy each chip and slowly savor it. Or try carrots and hummus. Make sure you replace the unhealthy food habit with a decent alternative that you actually like.

— *Get rid of your junk food stash.* Literally, just throw or give it all away. I have felt guilty throwing extra Halloween candy away in the past, so I kept a stash of it high in the pantry. So what did I do when I had a craving for it? I ate it! Now I give it all away to a group that sends it to our soldiers in the Middle East. They can enjoy it so my belly doesn't have to.

— *Modify your coffee-drinking habit.* If your habit is having four cups of coffee with cream and sugar every morning, try having two cups of coffee with steamed skim milk and a package of stevia.

Drink the coffee hot so you consume it more slowly and really enjoy it.

— *Don't skip breakfast.* If you are in the habit of skipping breakfast, be sure you understand the implications for your health and physiology. Skipping breakfast can negatively affect your mood, memory, and energy level throughout the day. Numerous studies have shown that people who have not eaten breakfast score lower on mental tests and report more fatigue.[2]

— *Replace sugary breakfast foods.* If you are in the habit of eating a sugary, unhealthy breakfast, try something hearty and filling that will make you feel satisfied until lunch, such as an over-easy egg with sautéed spinach and a little olive oil on a whole wheat English muffin. If you still crave sugar, have an organic blueberry waffle with a little real maple syrup.

— *Shop for healthy foods.* A big part of healthy eating starts at the grocery store and the foods you are in the habit of buying. If you usually get the same things every time you go shopping, including lots of processed and boxed food, you will have to retrain yourself to buy more fresh, whole foods and frozen healthy alternatives. Developing a shopping list based on healthy recipes can help immensely.

— *Avoid drinking soda.* Soda (or pop, as I call it) is full of sugar and calories that do not nourish you in any way whatsoever. If you've gotten in the habit of drinking more than one a day, see if you can cut back to one, or none, and substitute with flavored water or diet soda if you have to.

Solutions for Emotional Eating

From the time we are children, food is used to comfort, love, and sustain us. Some of my favorite childhood memories revolve around the delicious meals eaten in my grandmother's kitchen. I can still remember the amazing smells and the joy I felt consuming grandmother's homemade bread, macaroni and cheese, tomato soup, pot roast, molasses cookies, and a few Norwegian specialties. These were not culinary masterpieces, but they were made just for my brother, cousins, and me with such love. We reminisced about my grandma's cooking at her funeral with such fondness. She cooked comforting food to show us all how much she loved us, and it did make us feel so special.

It's no wonder that we eat to try to make ourselves feel better. We are wired and raised to believe that food can comfort us. In certain situations, it truly can. We've all been through a tough time and used food as a soothing balm. After the deaths of loved ones, people bring food to show their love and support. When we are utterly spent and exhausted from caring for a newborn baby, we might seek a comforting meal to give us a boost. However, when food is used to try to bandage up a broken life, it will never be enough, and it cannot heal you more than temporarily. The implications of using food to heal your life can be tragic to your health and waistline. For longer-term tough times, we need to discover healthier ways to comfort and soothe ourselves.

Here are a few suggestions for discovering alternatives to food for emotional sustenance:

— When you are craving a fatty takeout order after a tough day, try taking a walk to improve your mood and then ordering something fun but healthy for dinner instead.

— When you are feeling blue and can't pull yourself out of a funk, instead of eating something unhealthy, try watching a funny movie with a bowl of homemade salted popcorn.

— When you are feeling depressed and lonely, it can be hard to reach out to others. It may feel much easier to seek comfort in a container of ice cream. Instead, pick one person whom you trust and who makes you smile. Call that person and just say hello; then see where the conversation goes. Or just get out of the house and sit at a coffee shop with a magazine. Bring your baby in the stroller if you have to! I've met many new friends and one new nanny by chatting with complete strangers when I have been lonely during moves to new towns. The baby can be a huge icebreaker with other mothers, too.

— When I am feeling disconnected with my husband or I'm upset with a friend or family member, I find myself wanting to eat chocolate. I always think it will give me a little boost of joy. Now, I am a huge fan of dark chocolate and eat a few squares quite frequently, but when I am upset, I might eat the whole bar because I am seeking comfort. The fact is I rarely feel comforted after I eat the whole thing; rather, I feel disgusted with myself. If you are eating because you have discord in one of your life's key relationships, work on the relationship rather than trying to "eat it" better.

— If you eat more food or less healthy food when you are feeling stressed and anxious, try finding something else to "take the edge off." Maybe it's a yoga class or a walk with a close friend. A glass of wine while watching your favorite TV show can do wonders. Who needs the self-loathing that comes after overeating? Eating will only temporarily relieve the stress, while a healthy lifestyle can help you thrive through stress.

— After a particularly taxing day, instead of using food to relax and relieve you, try escaping for a while with a hot bath and a good book. You will come out feeling like a new woman.

Solutions for Social Eating

Social eating is my biggest weakness. One of my favorite things in life is sharing an incredible meal with special people. I love having friends over and engaging in conversation over good food. I always eat with reckless abandon during the holidays because I love the parties, fun drinks, and delectable treats. In fact, during one pregnancy, I gained seven pounds in five weeks over the holidays. Whoops! Subconsciously, I used to believe that by eating large quantities of food, I was showing love and respect to my hosts. Maybe that's a Midwestern thing? I regretted my gluttony every January when my pants felt too tight. Over time and with age, I have learned to rein myself in by eating only the treats I *really* love. I realize now that I was getting carried away in the festive mood and wasn't consciously enjoying half of what I was eating.

Women also like meals out with their girlfriends. Some of us get caught up in the fun of eating out and see it as an excuse to order whatever we're craving; then we feel compelled to finish the entire plate because everyone else has. When I was younger, I prided myself on eating whatever I wanted and not being overweight because I ran so much. As I've gotten older, I've learned I just can't do that anymore. Now I actually think about what I am going to order rather than ordering off the cuff. This has taken practice.

Here are a few suggestions for helping you reign in your social eating:

— I find if I've made a decision to eat well before I even leave my house, I tend to make better choices than when I make an impulsive, on-the-spot decision while the waiter is standing there. That's when I end up with a plate of steaming, gooey nachos and wonder what the heck I was thinking.

— Don't feel like you have to fit in with the crowd by ordering something you don't consider healthy if you are trying to watch your weight. Take time to really read the menu and find something that sounds truly wonderful to you. If you have to, ask to have it prepared in a healthier fashion (e.g., less cheese, more veggies, no bread, etc.).

— Don't go to a holiday party or any party without having a snack ahead of time. Self-control is that much harder to practice when you are starving.

— Don't obsess over food or talk about it all the time with your friends, but quietly make it known that you are watching your weight and are trying to make better choices. Good friends will respect that and will do what they can to support you.

— When you are invited to someone's home for dinner, bring a hostess gift, thank the person, and praise the food profusely— but don't feel like you have to eat gross quantities to get your point across.

Solutions for Mindless Eating

Everyone is guilty of eating mindlessly from time to time. I have consumed a bowl of popcorn the size of my head while watching an engrossing movie and then felt repulsed afterward. An issue closely tied to mindless eating is portion control. A good friend of mine told me that she scooped out a huge bowl of ice cream with the intention to share it with her husband. But as she watched her favorite show on TV, she looked down to discover that she had eaten every last bite—and she hadn't been aware enough to truly enjoy it.

We live in a culture of excess. Our portion sizes have gotten out of control, which makes mindless eating much more dangerous. If you only get the small bag of popcorn, or you only give yourself a normal portion of your favorite treat, you will be sure to really enjoy it rather than scarfing it down while focusing on something else. In reality, you can eat all of your very favorite foods even when you are watching your weight. The key is to be completely present while eating so you can savor every bite. When you eat this way, you will be satisfied with so much less. You won't feel deprived either.

Here are a few more tips to help you curb mindless eating:

— Do not eat in front of the TV unless you exercise portion control.

— When you can, sit down and eat meals as a family. Take the time to cook healthy, good-tasting food that you can eat slowly while enjoying conversation, and recognize when you are full. When you are full, stop eating and push your plate away as a signal to yourself that you are done.

— If you know you have a weakness for mindlessly eating a particular food, such as chips, candy, nuts, or buttered popcorn, don't buy it. It's so much easier if you just don't have it around to tempt you. If it's something you love, eat it as a special-occasion treat. If you still want to eat that food regularly, simply practice portion control.

— Be completely aware and present when you eat. By doing so, you will avoid mindless eating, you will savor what you're eating much more, and you will receive your body's signals that you've had enough.

— If you are at someone's house and he or she has bowls of chips and other treats sitting around, be sure not to sit right in front of the food so you can reduce the temptation to eat mindlessly.

Solutions for a Lack of Motivation to Exercise

Finding the motivation and energy to exercise after an exhausting night up feeding a fussy baby can be extraordinarily difficult. I know. I've been there! The solution is to just start moving. Even on our most tired days, some form of stretching, yoga, or walking will reinvigorate us at least a little.

Figuring out how to fit in exercise can also be intimidating to a new mom. You may ask yourself how you will squeeze it in between feedings, or wonder if it's safe to bring such a young baby to the gym's childcare, or worry that it is too sunny or hot in the stroller. I can tell you this—if it's important enough to you, you will discover and create solutions to address all of these concerns. The bigger issue is getting motivated to simply start moving.

Here are some creative ideas that you can implement to begin getting in some exercise:

— Schedule your workouts at the beginning of the week. Use the workout schedules from this book. (You can tear out or photocopy the master workout schedule at the end of each month's section.) Determine what you are going to do and how you are going to make it happen with the baby and other kids ahead of time. Check off each day as you accomplish the workouts. If you've got it written down, you will be much less likely to back out.

— Reward yourself when you meet your goals and complete all the workouts you have scheduled for the week. The reward might be a pedicure, a glass of wine, or a new workout top.

— Start walking with your stroller. When walking a few miles feels easy, try to jog a mile. One of the best cardio workouts you can get is running. If you decide you want running to be part of your regular workout routine, you need to make it as enjoyable as possible. Load interesting podcasts and upbeat music onto your iPhone or MP3 player. Get yourself the nicest jogging stroller that you can afford. Like I said, my double jogging stroller was quite an investment, but it was completely worth the freedom it brings to my life.

— Go to the library and pick out a new workout video to try at home each week. I have discovered some super fun, motivating, and effective workouts that I can do in my living room during naptime.

— If you live in a place that has inclement weather from time to time (which is almost everywhere), you should strongly consider joining a gym. Gyms offer numerous benefits, including socialization, a chance to meet new friends, the opportunity to try different and challenging classes, and a place to run or use the elliptical machine no matter what's going on outside. Many gyms offer great childcare that starts as early as six weeks. My children all started going to the gym at six weeks and generally just slept in their car seats the entire time. Most gyms also have great TVs so you can enjoy your favorite daytime shows while getting your body back in shape.

— Make plans to walk or jog with a friend. Having someone there to hold you accountable is extremely valuable. When my first child was born, I lived at a remote military installation with no childcare at the gym, but my girlfriend and I got together twice a week and practiced yoga from a book in her living room. The babies rolled around on a blanket or napped while we bonded for life on our yoga mats.

Nourishment: Do I Need to Take Vitamins and Supplements?

Do you feel energized and amazing every day? I wish I could say I did, but the truth is that there are stretches of time where I feel listless and lethargic, and I think most moms of small children feel the same way. During these times, I look at my life, and it's easy to see why. I generally eat very healthy, but lack of sleep and stress can still wreak havoc on my body. These are also the times I am most likely to forget to take my vitamins! As I get older and smarter, I have been more disciplined about taking my vitamins, and the effects have been very noticeable. I haven't been sick since implementing my regular vitamin regime.

Why wouldn't you take vitamins and supplements? They basically ensure that you are making up for the deficiencies in your diet, and they keep your body on an even keel despite the additional stress and sleep deprivation you might be experiencing. Here are the basic supplements that I, and most experts, recommend:

— *Multivitamin.* Definitely take a multivitamin. According to Dr. Oz, only one percent of a study group of three million people got enough of the essential vitamins their bodies needed for optimal health through diet alone.[3] Try to find a high-quality multivitamin that includes at least 100 percent of the 12 essential vitamins and minerals.

— *Iron.* I also recommend supplementing your diet with iron since you've just had a baby. According to the National Institutes of Health, a woman's iron needs go from 18 mg/day for ages 19 to 50, up to 27 mg/day if you are pregnant, and 9 mg/day if you are nursing (less is required because you are generally not getting your period while nursing).[4] Iron supplements are best absorbed on an empty stomach or after eating foods high in vitamin C, such as citrus fruits or tomatoes. I've been anemic, and it feels as though you have lead running through your veins; you are constantly exhausted. If you have felt strangely tired for an extended period of time, get a blood test for iron. Also, people who are tired all the time are frequently deficient in vitamin B12, which is a well-known energy-boosting vitamin.

— *Calcium, Magnesium, and Vitamin D.* Fifty-five percent of Americans over the age of 50 have osteoporosis; 80 percent of them are women. It's hard to get enough calcium if you aren't a big milk drinker, so why not take a supplement? Dr. Oz recommends that women take 600 mg of calcium with 400 mg of magnesium and 1,000 IU of vitamin D, all together, for maximum effectiveness.[5]

— *Fish Oil.* Fish oil pills contain omega-3 fatty acids, which are proven to lower your risk of heart attack and in some studies have reduced rates of depression. One thing to watch for is where the fish comes from. Try to make sure it is a source that minimizes the potential for mercury and PCB contamination from fish swimming in polluted water. Dr. Oz recommends 600–1000 mg of the omega-3 fatty acid DHA.[6]

If you want to implement an easy and fairly inexpensive measure for living a more healthful and energized life, consider taking these basic supplements. There are many other useful supplements and additional vitamins that you can consider; however this list is a great place to start and should keep you very healthy and feeling good.

Fitness: Making Exercise a Priority

In this third week, we are going to really start focusing on exercise. The challenge is finding time between feedings, naps, and chores to get out for a walk or jog, or even to the gym. With a little planning, however, you can start making your workouts a priority.

There are many things that come up each day that can oust your workout, and some of them are legitimate. The key is to differentiate between real reasons and simple excuses. There are days when you haven't gotten enough sleep and feel too tired to get off the couch. Real sleep deprivation is a problem, as we've discussed here! In that case, it is your judgment call. Ideally, you could fit in both a short nap and a brief workout; but some days, sleep simply wins, and that's okay. At other times, you might just be feeling lazy and a little tired, and a bit of walking in the fresh air might give you the energy boost you need to get through the day.

Try to do some form of exercise six days this week. Select workouts that fit into your schedule, preferably including two strength workouts and two or more cardio workouts (see the suggested schedule below). Do the best that you can. I know it's tough when you're sleep deprived and busy, but I will stress that working out gets easier with time and makes you feel more energetic and happy overall!

Week 3 Workout Schedule

Monday	Tuesday	Wednesday	Thursday	Friday	Saturday	Sunday
30-minute walk or 20-minute jog	15 minutes strength	1-hour walk or cardio class at gym	15 minutes strength	30-minute walk or cardio class at gym	Yoga or Pilates class	Rest

Core-Rocking Workout

This strength workout is one you can do at home without any equipment. It will help you start strengthening and toning your core muscles, which were stretched and weakened during pregnancy and childbirth. Go through the entire series of exercises three times after a warm-up of walking, jogging in place, or dancing around the house!

1. *Modified Plank.* Start by lifting your body up on your forearms and toes, keeping your body as straight as possible, as shown. Keep your spine neutral and your feet about an inch apart. Work your way up to holding this pose for a minute or more, breathing deeply the entire time.

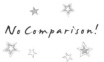
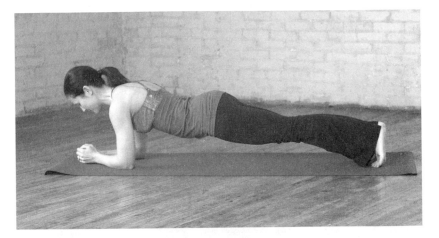

Modified Plank, presented by Anne, hot mama of Kaden and Jennika

2. *Side Plank.* Start in a plank position on your hands and the balls of your feet. Shift your body to your left side, moving onto the outside edge of your left foot, and stack your right foot directly on top. Support the weight of your body on the outer left foot and left hand, and stretch your right arm up to the ceiling. Try to align your body into one long line from your heels to the top of your head. Hold for 30 seconds on each side.

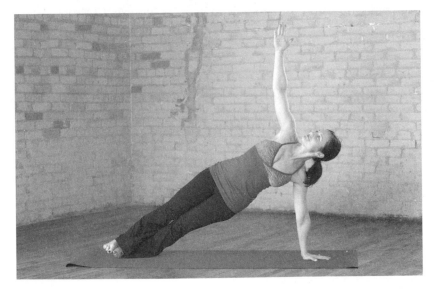

3. *Side Plank with a Twist.* Start on your left side with elbow on the floor, directly under your shoulder and hips stacked. Lift your hips up, creating a straight line from your head to heels, and extend your right arm up to the ceiling. Next, scoop your right arm from an upward position to under your body, rotating your upper body. Hold for a breath and then return your arm straight up and repeat ten times.

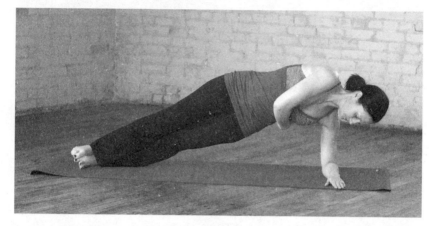

4. *Superman.* Lie on your stomach, and raise both your arms and your legs a few inches off the floor, until you feel your lower back working. Hold for three deep breaths. Repeat 12 times.

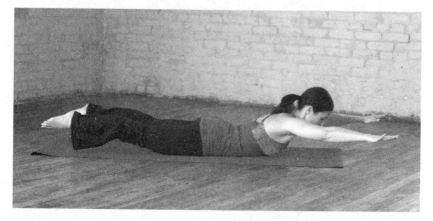

5. *Balancing Table Pose.* Start on your hands and knees, and with an inhale, lift your left leg straight back, and also lift your right arm straight out from the shoulder, parallel to the floor. Point your toes toward the back wall while stretching and reaching your fingers toward the wall in front of you. Feel the muscles in your back working, and hold for five breaths. Then switch to your right leg and left arm.

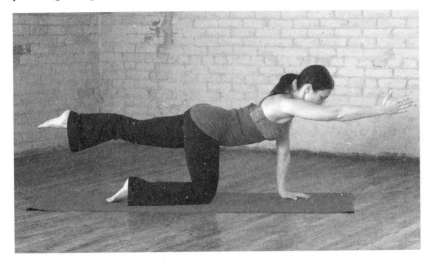

Sanity Saver: Napping

I know I talked extensively about sleep in Week 1, but we are going to revisit this precious act of self-love. When you have that heavy feeling in your body, as though you just need to lie down, please promise me you will do it. Nap when the baby naps, and if you have to entertain your older children, a 30- or 45-minute video will not kill them.

A 20- to 30-minute power nap should be most beneficial for you. Human sleep patterns occur in five stages. Naps should take you from Stage 1 (when you are just drifting off) into Stage 2 (when your brain activity slows); then you will wake up feeling rejuvenated and alert. If you allow yourself to go into the deeper sleep stages (3 and 4), you could wake up feeling more tired and groggy than when you started. If I am unable to sleep, I have found that just lying in bed for 20 minutes makes me feel refreshed.

Stages of Sleep

Stage 1. Stage 1 sleep is light sleep, when you are drifting in and out and are easily awakened.

Stage 2. During stage 2 sleep, eye movements stop and brain waves slow significantly.

Stage 3. This is the first stage of deep sleep, where brain waves oscillate between slow delta waves and faster waves.

Stage 4. Stage 4 sleep is the second stage of deep sleep, signified by slow delta brain waves. It is difficult to wake someone up in stage 3 or 4 sleep.

REM. Rapid eye movement (REM) sleep is the sleep stage in which dreaming occurs. Your eyes move rapidly, and your muscles become immobile. Heart rate and blood pressure increase.

Proven benefits of napping include the following:

- Reducing stress
- Boosting your immune system
- Restoring alertness
- Enhancing performance
- Reducing mistakes
- Having fewer accidents

I also want to point out that napping has some fabulous psychological benefits, as well. A nap for a mom can be seen as a little escape and an indulgent break. After letting our bodies and brains rest completely, we can come back to our lives feeling much more on an even keel. You may not need to nap every day, but when the opportunity presents itself and it feels like the right thing to do, please indulge!

Affirmation for the Week

I was created just the way I am for a reason. I am beautiful and unique, and have gifts to offer this world in a way that nobody else can. When I take care of my mind, spirit, and body, my outer beauty will reflect my inner light and magnificence. Becoming the very best version of myself is the best way I can live a confident, whole, and joyful life.

I will eat in a way that honors my body and makes me feel alive. Becoming conscious of my choices and of what I am putting in my mouth shows my body love and respect. Nourishing and moving my body will help me have energy to really enjoy my life. Becoming more aware of my eating and exercise pitfalls will help me make better decisions and choices. I am capable of eating well and doing the things necessary to feel and look my best.

★◻★

New Normalcy

"Normal day, let me be aware of the treasure you are. Let me learn from you, love you, bless you before you depart. Let me not pass you by in quest of some rare and perfect tomorrow. Let me hold you while I may, for it may not always be so."

—MARY JEAN IRON

I once heard a fellow Air Force wife talking about how she dealt with raising six children, one of them a nursing newborn. I listened with serious intent, since at the time I had no children, and any child seemed like a major undertaking. She said, "Life with all these children is just my new normal. I have to be very organized and really just have to always keep moving, but my children know the drill and the older ones pretty much take care of themselves. Most of the work comes from the youngest two, and the older kids actually lighten my load and help out." I felt that I had something to learn from this woman. What I noticed most about her was that she was very relaxed and just seemed to enjoy life. Nothing seemed to fluster her. She had gotten to a place where she was truly comfortable and happy in her life, and she honestly enjoyed each of her six kids.

Why do I share this woman's story? Because she highlighted something that really stood out to me. Her life with her children was her new normal. She and her husband completely adapted. They still went out on date nights every few weeks, at a minimum, and they tried to put their marriage first. She claimed that the kids had mostly enhanced their relationship. "Oh, yes!" she exclaimed.

"There have been moments that were horrible with multiple sick kids and screaming, colicky babies, but it's all been worth it." Here is the kicker: Her kids were amazing. They were the most polite, helpful, loving children.

Having six children is certainly not for me, but if this woman can thrive while raising that many, we can all do it, too. I know plenty of moms of four and five children who also do it beautifully. It gives me hope that the rest of us can thrive with one, two, or three kids. We simply need to embrace this new normal.

Mourning a Loss

We all have moments when we mourn aspects of our "pre-child" lives, such as spending money how we wanted, focusing our financial resources on our wardrobes and fun trips with our husbands, spontaneous fun, and carefree partying with late nights out. That's completely normal! Just don't spend too much time in mourning. Life is a series of phases or seasons, and we've moved into a beautiful new one. We can still have those fun shopping trips, occasional child-free vacations with our husbands, and crazy party nights, but they will just be far less frequent. The upside is that you appreciate those opportunities much more than you did in your pre-baby years. You should savor every minute and not take these occasions for granted, since they don't occur every week anymore.

Many of us miss our pre-baby bodies, too. I recently saw a photo of myself at the beach in my early 20s and thought, *Wow, did I have a great stomach!* The funny thing is that I don't remember thinking I looked that good back then. My belly is okay now, but three babies can do a little semi-permanent morphing to the midsection. In 20 years, we are all going to look at photos of ourselves now and think, *Dang, I looked fabulous back then.* There are more important things than a perfect belly. We need to love our bodies, take the best care of them we can, and then move on with our lives.

The point of this discussion is that our lives have changed forever. We are now responsible for other human beings, and they need to be our priorities, in general. This is an absolute blessing and honor, and we need to try our best to see it as such. Sure, there are going to be moments, even whole days, when we miss the freedom and ease of our earlier years. But savor these memories and feel confident that you have lived each season of your life to the fullest.

Here are a few ways to make sure that you are still having enough fun, excitement, and selfish moments to minimize mourning over your pre-baby life:

— Make sure you are still doing what you can financially to dress in a way that makes you feel cute and attractive. You are still you, and you want your clothes to express who you are.

— Save up money for an occasional splurge. Is there a pair of sunglasses or a gorgeous handbag that you noticed in a magazine? Cut out the picture and put it up somewhere you will see it regularly. Save for as long as you need to in order to purchase it. If it's something that you think is absolutely beautiful, do what you can to make it yours.

— Make date nights a priority. I will say it countless times throughout this book, but if you are married, then your relationship with your husband is the rock that your family is built around. If you aren't taking the time to nurture this critical relationship, you might seriously regret it down the road. Your kids are important, but your relationship with your husband is the reason you decided to create a family in the first place. Keep this relationship strong.

— Go out on the town. Take a shower, fix your hair, and put on the best outfit you have. Get out. Meet some girlfriends for dinner or have a martini with your best friend. Go dancing. Just because you're a mom doesn't mean you're not fun and hot! Moms can dance. Trust me.

Getting into a Rhythm

One of the things I recommend highly for all mamas is getting into a new rhythm and routine in your life. Letting the baby dictate your activities might work best when the little one is a few days or weeks old, but there comes a point when it's healthiest for all of you to get into a regular schedule.

Routines can help with many areas of your life, such as making sure you get your exercise in every day, ensuring a daily shower, getting your baby to sleep regularly, and keeping your home life more organized. I write about this a lot because it's not my natural way of being, but when I get my children and myself on a routine, we all do so much better. Babies and children like to know what to expect, and I think adults thrive on routine nearly as much as kids do.

Here are a few areas of your life where routines can do wonders.

Morning

Any mom knows that getting out the door in the morning can be a little hectic, and sometimes downright hellish. There are days when getting my oldest child up, dressed, and out the door for school is the most stressful event of my day. On the most challenging days, kids melt down and moms want to have a breakdown.

Establishing a morning routine can make the start of your day so much more pleasant. Regular activities might include relaxing at home with the baby, a newspaper, and a cup of coffee; or laying out your older kids' clothes and packing lunches the night before to make the morning run more smoothly. One thing that I, and countless other moms, can attest to is that children do not like to be rushed. Rushing them is counterproductive and actually makes them slow down. Babies simply won't be rushed, so you've just got to make sure you have the time to meet their needs. Otherwise, you will be late.

My personal routine starts with some quiet time before the family wakes up; I enjoy hot coffee, inspirational reading, meditation, and prayer. Sometimes I have to do this while snuggling with a sleepy little one, but it's still my time. I do what I can to get this precious quiet time on a majority of mornings, but some mornings I am just too exhausted and need sleep more. When I do get up early and have this special time, I start the day centered, grateful, and much more present and peaceful. I recommend having a chunk of time like this every day, whether it's first thing or any other time.

Regarding my kids, I have learned that first of all, things go more smoothly when they've had a good night of sleep. I have also learned the hard way that you need to make sure you have a good hour to get ready before you have to be anywhere. The routine I established with my firstborn when she was about two years old is that she wakes up and comes to find me in my special chair having my meditation time.

Breakfast will go most efficiently if you have easy-to-make, delicious, healthy things ready to prepare. I feed my kids in their PJs to protect their clothes from spills and other breakfast madness. After breakfast, we get dressed in clothes we picked out the night before. If I don't pick clothes out the night before, I give my children two options only. Some of our most stressful, argumentative mornings have involved an outfit that my daughter adamantly wanted to wear that I just could not let her (because it was simply too hideous or completely weather inappropriate, such as a sundress and flip-flops on a freezing cold day!). Sometimes, if the outfit isn't too awful, I just let her wear what she thinks looks good. It's an act of self-expression, and really, what's the harm? Most moms understand.

I often put my exercise clothes on first thing in the morning. I will elaborate on my reasoning in the next section, but my morning routine includes working out during naptime for my baby and toddler and then showering. On the days I go to work, I have to wake up a little earlier and try to get in the shower very first thing, even before quiet time; otherwise, it starts to feel impossible to fit it all in and still look decent.

Do you take your baby to childcare? If so, pack up her diaper bag or whatever else she might need the night before. It's not fun to rush around trying to find a missing pacifier when running a few minutes behind schedule.

Figure out what would bring you joy in the morning, and start your day that way. How can you best set the tone for your day? Think of where you have the biggest roadblocks and stressors, and then brainstorm ways to make them go more smoothly.

Exercise

The best way to make sure you exercise nearly every day is by getting into a routine. Once you get in the routine of jogging with your girlfriend every Tuesday or hitting an amazing yoga class on Friday, you will be sad to miss it. Getting into an exercise routine means making this crucial activity an important part of your life.

A great way to establish a routine is to sit down on Sunday and put your workouts into a day planner or on a calendar. Photocopy each month's workout schedule and post it where you will see it regularly. Set dates with people so you can't back out. Look at the gym's schedule and the weather forecast. On the days when you know you will be busy, plan to do a shorter workout video or weight routine from home. Once these classes or workouts are written down or put into your electronic calendar, do everything you can to make sure they happen. Exercise needs to be important to you; otherwise, you will easily find reasons to let it slip.

Housekeeping and Errands

Get a housecleaner every week. The end. Oh, if it were only so easy! The key to maintaining an organized and Zen-like house is to create simple routines and systems for picking up, laundry, doing deeper cleaning, and running errands.

I did have a housecleaning service when I worked, and it was fabulous. I hope to have one again someday! If you can afford it, I highly recommend having someone help you with the deep cleaning every week or so. You will still have plenty to do, but at least you won't spend so much of your precious free time scrubbing. Nowadays, I clean my big old house on a rotating schedule. There is no way I can take the time to clean the entire house at once, unless I neglect my children for hours at a time.

I have polled countless busy moms who have particularly beautiful and organized homes to learn just how they do it, and they all have a variation of the same routine. Either they have a housecleaner, or they have established a routine to clean a little of their house every day. For example, every Monday they dust all the surfaces in the house, every Tuesday they do the bathrooms, Wednesdays they clean the floors, Thursdays they scrub the kitchen, etc. This way, cleaning the entire house doesn't seem quite so taxing.

I have also found that if I do a little laundry every day, it is much less overwhelming. When I worked outside the home, I used to save it all up for the weekends. When I'd finally get it all piled up and ready to start washing, it about made me sick to my stomach to see the massive volume that had collected in just a week. I also recommend that you record your favorite shows and catch up on them while folding laundry—it makes the task seem a bit more enjoyable!

Here are few other useful tips:

— Lower your standards, at least a little. Before having kids, you may have had a perfectly spotless house. That feels peaceful and fabulous, but it can make you crazy to maintain when you have babies and children. If your house is a mess but you are exhausted, take care of yourself first, with a nap or a little down time. A little messiness never killed anyone. Always put your wellness and important relationships before cleanliness!

— Listen to fun or inspirational podcasts or Hay House Radio live on your smartphone while you clean.

— Clean as you go while you are cooking. For example, wipe down the counters and put dishes in the dishwasher while the water is boiling or the meal is baking, so the messes are cleaned up in smaller, more digestible bits.

— Teach your children to pick up after themselves at a very early age, and give them easy places to put their toys. I have friends who have put labeled bins on their shelves to really keep things organized. I don't take it that far, but if that might work for you, you should try it.

Grocery Shopping and Cooking

One of the biggest demands on many moms' time each week is grocery shopping and preparing meals. Unfortunately, around dinnertime is the fussiest time of the day for many babies, making it tough to prepare for dinner. Getting into a routine and having easy, yummy, nourishing recipes with all the ingredients on hand will make this time of day substantially less stressful.

During the weeks when I am organized and take the time to plan meals and develop shopping lists, cooking dinner becomes more fun. I can even get my husband to cook occasionally if we have all of the ingredients in the house. I cannot stand getting to the end of a long day and trying to magically produce a decent meal from the random things in the cupboard. I have had very mixed luck with my last-minute, hodgepodge creations!

Establish a routine for grocery shopping. The night before, sit down with a cooking magazine (I love *Cooking Light* and *Food & Wine*) or a single cookbook, and pick three or four recipes for the week. Mark those recipes, and then create a shopping list for the ingredients. Lay the list out so that as other things come to mind (such as toilet paper and toothpaste), they can be easily added. Another great way to develop a weekly meal plan is using the Epicurious iPhone application. It is easy to find recipes that are delicious and highly rated. Then you can automatically create a shopping list based on the recipes you've selected, complete with check boxes, which you can have right in your hand at the grocery store. An additional awesome source of fun, new recipes is the multitude of fabulous cooking blogs. Some have stunning photos that will inspire you to try new recipes.

I also purchase organic frozen pizzas or another incredibly easy dinner option for one night a week (or more, depending on what I've got going on). One of the nights you can plan on cleaning out the refrigerator by eating leftovers. We also always eat out or order takeout at least one night a week.

Napping

After polling numerous moms, the one area of their lives where they find routine to be the most beneficial is naptime. Babies thrive on routine, and it's very healthy for kids to be on a regular schedule. Putting your baby down for naps at the same times every day will ensure he or she is getting enough sleep, will help reduce fussiness, and will allow you to have a chunk of time for yourself. Naps will help you get your own nap, if that's what you need, or a workout, some cleaning, or attention to a creative project. Developing a nap routine might take a little effort, but once it is established, your life will improve dramatically.

Creative and Intellectual Time

Creative and intellectual stimulation are crucial for anyone to live a well-balanced life, but especially for moms. Taking time to nourish this side of yourself will make you a happier woman and a more balanced person. Most women I know, myself included, do not generally make creative time a scheduled priority. This has changed for me recently, and it has been positively life altering.

We all have something inside us that needs to be brought to life, whether it's writing, painting, or photography. If you don't know what your creative gift is, keep paying attention. Maybe your outlet is trying new recipes and cooking amazing meals on occasion or reading an inspirational book. Maybe you just want to take the time to learn about technology or politics.

Creative expression is one of the easiest things to let go by the wayside as a mother. But taking the time to nurture your intellect and your creative spirit is one of the key ingredients to not losing yourself to motherhood.

Bedtime

Babies and children need activities that signal various daily events. Develop a soothing, relaxing bedtime routine that signals to your child that it's time to wind down. Perhaps start with taking a bath and putting on pajamas, then reading a few books and singing a song. Even babies thrive on knowing what to expect. As these regular activities occur, they start to prepare for bed; after time, when you lay them in their crib, they will simply go to sleep without a fuss. Time this routine so that your baby is nice and sleepy but not overly exhausted by the time you put him or her in bed. Over-exhaustion has a strange effect on children and often makes them wired—so they have a difficult time shutting down and falling asleep.

One of the benefits of having a bedtime routine is that it helps when other people must put your child to bed. When a family member or a babysitter is watching my children, I explain or write down the bedtime process, including the time it starts, so that things feel somewhat normal to my kids. It helps them feel the comfort of their routine, so they can drift off to sleep just like they normally do.

Nourishment: Your Relationship with Food

Were you surprised by the results of the quiz you took in Week 3 about your eating habits? I was. I knew I was a social eater, but as it turns out, I can also be an emotional or mindless eater. I think most of us fall into different overeating pitfalls from time to time! The trick is to be aware of these human weaknesses and to develop effective solutions to avoid them.

Have you ever taken the time to really think about your relationship with food? Do you eat in a way that is mostly good for your health? Do you enjoy the food you eat? I have worked with many people who say they sometimes finish a meal and then realize they weren't present enough to really enjoy it. They look down at the end and think, *Wow—did I just eat all that?*

When you indulge in rich or unhealthy food, you do not have to feel guilty. Delicious food is one of the great joys of living on this earth! Just make sure you are making it worth the extra calories. By that, I mean relish each bite. Eat slowly, and enjoy the smell and texture. Indulging in meals like this should not happen every day, so that when it happens, the experience should be appreciated and savored.

Everyday meals should also taste wonderful, while being nourishing and healthy. Eat meals with that will benefit you in more ways than one. Meals are social, bringing families and friends together around a table. They are an emotional experience and are a wonderful part of enjoying life. However, we need to identify if we have let food control us in ways that are not positive.

The best advice I can give you about having a healthy relationship with food, meaning being able to stay fit while enjoying good meals, is to be present and aware. Being aware of your potential to overeat doesn't mean you have to avoid certain foods or situations entirely; just try to exercise more control over yourself and your actions. You are the one in command of your nutrition and health. If what you are currently doing is not working for you, you need to do some self-evaluation until the way you eat is in alignment with the true you!

Fitness: Your Progress So Far

I wish I could sit down with each of you to talk about how the first month of getting your body back after having a baby has been going. Has it been enjoyable? Frustrating? Rewarding? I promise you this: The first month is the most difficult and painful. Things will really start to feel more enjoyable as you get in better shape.

I will never forget the first few runs after having each baby. Running is usually soothing and therapeutic for me; I was not used to being in pain and miserable while running. Those first runs were just that—miserable. Slowly but surely, I plodded along, confident that it would eventually get easier. A few weeks later, I realized that I could do my three-mile loop without too much suffering. Hang in there; running, or any other exercise that you stick to, will get easier.

Are you noticing a difference in your fitness level? Are you able to exercise a little longer or harder? Can you feel your clothes fitting better? The improvements in your body and fitness level may be slow in coming, but they will come. If it helps you feel more accomplished, the next week or two is the right time to start tracking your body measurements or weight on a weekly basis. You might also track your workouts on paper or on your computer. Otherwise, continue to push your body during your workouts just to see what you are capable of. Add a few minutes to your daily walk, do an extra repetition, or lift slightly heavier weights. You are going to start liking the results, both in the way you feel and the way you look.

The workout schedule for Week 4 features a five-minute increase for the strength workouts on Tuesday and Thursday. Remember that this is an ideal workout schedule, and you can add or subtract time and modify the strenuousness based on how you are feeling and your fitness level.

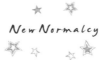
Week 4 Workout Schedule

Monday	Tuesday	Wednesday	Thursday	Friday	Saturday	Sunday
30-minute walk or 20-minute jog	20 minutes strength	1-hour walk, 30-minute jog, or cardio class at gym	20 minutes strength	30-minute walk, 20-minute jog, or cardio class at gym	Yoga or Pilates class	Rest

Cardio Blast Circuit

It is time to get out of your comfort zone! If you have been walking or jogging and feel like you're getting in good shape, try a half-hour walk followed by this cardio blast circuit. You can do this workout on busy days when you are at home or in conjunction with a strength workout.

1. *Jog in Place.* Jog in place for five minutes, or even jog around your house. Use a watch or phone to time yourself.

2. *Jumping Jacks.* Do jumping jacks for three minutes straight. Then march in place for a minute.

3. *Burpees with a Push-up.* Start by standing, and then drop into a squat with your hands on the ground. Jump back to a plank position and do one push-up. Jump back to the squat position, and stand back up—jump up to the sky if you've got it in you! That completes one burpee. Repeat ten times.

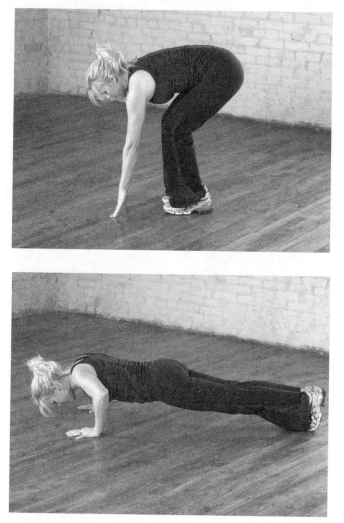

Burpees with a Push-up, presented by Tyanne, hot mama of Kate and Ava.

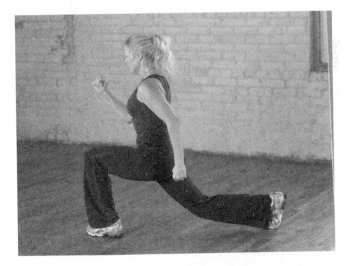

4. *Jump Switch Lunges*. Start with a little hop forward into a deep lunge with your right leg, until your thigh is parallel to the floor. Jump up and switch legs, using your arms for momentum. Repeat 15 times.

5. *Squat Jumps.* Start by standing with your feet about shoulder-width apart, arms at your sides. Do a regular squat until your thighs are parallel to the floor. Then jump up as high and as explosively as you can, using your arms and reaching for the ceiling. Land as gently as you can, then lower back into a squat position to start the next repetition. Repeat 10 to 15 times.

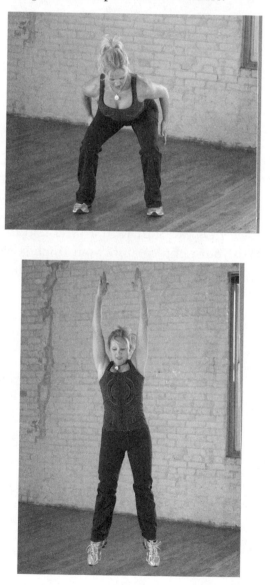

After a heart-thumping cardio workout, it's always a good idea to cool down with some marching in place and stretching for at least ten minutes.

Sanity Saver: Meditation and Prayer

While having coffee with my sister-in-law recently, I asked her, "When do you feel most beautiful?" I thought she would tell me when her husband gave her a nice compliment, after a new haircut, or when wearing a gorgeous new outfit. Her reply took me by surprise. She responded that she felt most beautiful when she was spiritually focused and centered, when she took the time to be still. She said that when she felt close to God, she felt beautiful from the inside—and then the other areas of her life, such as her relationship with her husband and the way she mothers her children, just fell into place.

Meditation and prayer are two of the most powerful ways to create a calm center in your life. Meditation is essentially any practice that calms the mind by engaging in breathing and sitting peacefully in reflection. Some practices include trying to empty the mind of any thoughts, while others include thought observation and a focus on breath. There is even meditation that can be done while walking! Three common types of meditation are:

— *Mindfulness Meditation.* This style of meditation involves sitting quietly in a comfortable position and concentrating on an object, a process, or what is happening around you. The key is that you are aware of your feelings and the thoughts that come into your mind, which you are to observe but not judge. I've learned two useful methods for observing thoughts and then letting them go without judgment: 1) View your thoughts as clouds passing in the sky. Watch a thought come into your mind, observe it, and let it float out. 2) Another mindfulness practice I like is visualizing my thoughts as though they are being written on a chalkboard in my mind. After I've considered the thought, I erase it and sit in silence until another one comes.

— *Breathing Meditation.* This type of meditation is as easy as it sounds. Just sit and breathe, focusing all of your attention on the breath coming in and going out. I often do this in counts of three or six, meaning I breathe in for three counts, hold my breath for three counts, and then let it out for six counts. This meditation is so easy, and it calms the mind and entire body very quickly. It can be done anywhere, any time you need to relax your mind and body (for example, before blowing up at your kids!). There are many breathing techniques, which you can learn through guided meditation and then practice on your own.

— *Empty Mind Meditation.* During this type of meditation, the goal is to empty your mind of any thoughts and let it simply rest. When this is done successfully, a deep sense of peace and calm will take over. This meditation requires a quiet, comfortable room with no distractions, so you can truly allow your mind to become still. For me, this one only works if I have done some other meditation or yoga first. It's tough for a busy, overtasked mind to become "empty" right away!

Meditation Basics

Dedicate at least 10 to 30 minutes every day to being still and quiet. Start by trying out a variety of recorded guided meditations (in which a person directs you through the meditation process), and then decide which methods work best for you. Meditation is personal, and it can change every day.

Go to a special place to meditate, at a time you know you will have a few minutes of uninterrupted quiet.

Relax your body and start breathing.

Once your mind is very still and your body is relaxed, just observe your thoughts. Let them come and go, never judging them.

Let tension and negative feelings drain from your body. Then fill your body with light and love as you breathe in. Pay attention to where your body is tight, and remind yourself to "let go" of stress.

When you're finished, go out into the world filled with peace, and spread your loving energy!

An important thing to remember is that there is no wrong way to meditate. Some mornings my meditation and prayer run together, and I only get five minutes in before one of my kids interrupts my peace . . . but it still helps me immensely! Many women are intimidated by meditation and attempt it by just sitting down and trying not to think. Most moms I know will go into a state of "monkey mind" pretty quickly if they do this. Thoughts will start running rampant, about the cupcakes that were supposed to be baked last night, now necessitating a stop at the store; the credit card bill that needs to be paid; or an argument from the night before . . . the possibilities are endless. With practice, this inner chatter will subside.

Though practiced for centuries, meditation is often seen as far out and New Age. The health benefits, both physical and psychological, are quickly making fans of Western physicians. Meditation is free and can be done anywhere (although not always at any time if you are a mom with children at home). Meditation takes some practice, but the wide range of benefits is compelling. They include improvements in conditions such as allergies, anxiety, asthma, cancer, depression, fatigue, heart disease, high blood pressure, insomnia, and substance abuse.[1] Studies show that meditation even lowers cortisol levels, elevated by stress, in the blood.[2] Meditators are also shown to have better overall mental health, including superior concentration, memory, and productivity—three of the top complaint areas of women raising children![3] One statistic presented in the *International Journal of Neuroscience* that really caught my eye is that meditation has been shown to slow aging. Results indicated that study participants who had meditated for 5 years or more were an average of 12 years younger, physically and mentally, than their chronological age.[4] Within a few years, I will be "back in my 20s." I'm sold . . . love it!

People often think that prayer is only for the devout and religious. I believe prayer is for anyone who strives to be more spiritual. Studies have shown many positive implications related to health and longevity, similar to the effects of medication in some cases, in people who pray.[5] Some scientific research indicates that prayer is effective and influences outcomes. I use my prayer time to ask God and the universe to grant me abundance, peace, and love. It is an opportunity to express gratitude for all of the blessings in my life and ask for things and experiences that I desire. During some really tough times, I went into my prayer thinking I had little to be grateful for. Once I began praying, a multitude of blessings would flood my mind . . . simple things, such as a safe place to live, a warm bed, and a healthy family.

When you're lucky, you can thank God for little hands to hold, people to love, and people who love you. My favorite prayer is one for others; I send them love, healing, energy, and whatever they happen to need at the time, no matter where they are. I spend the most time on my husband and children; then I pray for my entire family and my dearest friends, whoever pops into my mind. An amazing combination is meditation followed by prayer. Even if I get my mind calm and peaceful for five minutes before I pray, the effect is dramatic. The thoughts flow, and my deepest needs and desires start surfacing. People in my life start entering my mind, and I know they need my love, prayer, and positive energy.

Affirmation for the Week

Life as a mother is certainly an adjustment, but a beautiful one. Children are bound to bring major changes to my life, but with a little flexibility and a lot of organization, the transition into motherhood will feel "meant to be." My life has been enriched and enhanced by my sweet baby more than I could have imagined. Yes, my life before my baby was fabulous; but it was not as rewarding or rich as it is now.

Routine is valuable for both my baby and me, and it will help me feel more balanced and peaceful. I will create a routine that works best for my family, one that ensures that I have time to care for myself and helps me meet my primary needs first—so that I am better able to love and serve my family. I will remember that children thrive when life is calm and they know what to expect, so routine will only foster a sense of comfort for them, too.

★✦★

Month 1 Workout Schedule

	Monday	Tuesday	Wednesday	Thursday	Friday	Saturday	Sunday
Week 1	30-minute walk	15 minutes strength	45-minute walk or low-impact cardio class at gym	15 minutes strength	30-minute walk or low-impact cardio class at gym	Yoga or Pilates class	Rest
Week 2	30-minute walk	15 minutes strength	45-minute walk or low-impact cardio class at gym	15 minutes strength	30-minute walk or low-impact cardio class at gym	Yoga or Pilates class	Rest
Week 3	30-minute walk or 20-minute jog	15 minutes strength	1-hour walk or cardio class at gym	15 minutes strength	30-minute walk or cardio class at gym	Yoga or Pilates class	Rest
Week 4	30-minute walk or 20-minute jog	20 minutes strength	1-hour walk, 30-minute jog, or cardio class at gym	20 minutes strength	30-minute walk, 20-minute jog, or cardio class at gym	Yoga or Pilates class	Rest

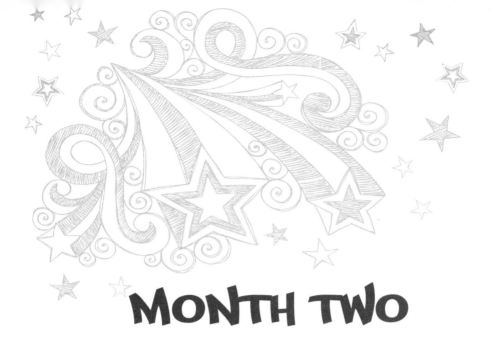

MONTH TWO

I hope that the first month of this program was enjoyable and that you are now getting into a beautiful rhythm that works well for you and your baby. Your fitness level should be increasing as your energy levels begin to soar. During the second month, we will discuss how to organize your mind and life in a way that makes things run smoothly for all. Relationships can be impacted by the arrival of a baby, but with a little effort and love, these connections can remain strong and even be enhanced. Motherhood is one of the most important roles you will ever have, but it doesn't define you. Being a mom is such a powerful and life-changing experience that it just might propel you to be a more confident woman—one who follows her dreams!

★ ◆ ★

Under Control

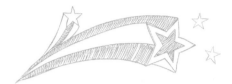

"Never mistake motion for action."

— ERNEST HEMINGWAY

Many women realize they are control freaks only after they become mothers. We don't realize it before because our lives are as calm and organized as we want them to be. Then . . . these tiny, helpless, needy creatures come into our lives to let us know we are not always in control. That can be tough to take!

Before kids, I would never have labeled myself a control freak. In fact, I've always thought I was a super laid-back, peaceful, go-with-the-flow kind of girl. Turns out, I was able to be that way because my life was completely under my command. I have the ability to be incredibly relaxed when my house is organized and my life feels under control. I've now discovered that when my house and life feel completely out of control, I do, too. In talking to dozens of women about this, I have realized I am not alone.

I am just sitting down to write again after picking up my house. I realized I was sitting down to write about organization when my own living space was fairly disastrous, with toys and books scattered about. The sense that overcame me was "disorganization." How could I write about organization when my own house was a crazy mess? So I am back again to offer tips that I have learned through trial and error myself, or gathered from countless women throughout the country.

Organize Your Thoughts

Before we can organize our lives, we need to make sure our minds are collected and clear. When our thoughts are scattered and disorganized, we can feel like the rest of our life is disjointed and lacks something essential.

Many women I talk with complain of obsessive thinking. The National Science Foundation claims that the average person has 12,000 unique thoughts per day, while a more active thinker has around 55,000 thoughts. I have also heard statistics that many women have upwards of 70,000 thoughts per day. Regardless of the actual number, the point is that our brains are working nonstop.

How many of our thoughts are beneficial? How many of us have minds that constantly churn, sometimes without a lot of control or input from us? The more we evolve, the better we can control our minds and use them to our benefit. Many of our thoughts have no purpose, and even worse, are assumptions, worries, and wastes of energy. How much of our brainpower is squandered by worrying about things that will never happen or that happened in the past?

Worrying causes our body to feel and experience stress, which has its own negative implications. Motherhood brings a whole new set of things to worry about, many of which are tough to overcome when we are naturally so protective of our children. We have to remember that worrying cannot keep anyone safe or change any situation for the better. Our bodies cannot differentiate between worry and an actually dangerous situation. Therefore, the body's natural fight-or-flight response kicks in, causing increases in stress hormones and the damaging effects of stress on our health. Many moms live in a constant state of anxiety, largely due to ongoing worry and constantly disorganized and uncontrolled thinking.

By obsessively worrying and stewing over your thoughts, you are unknowingly activating a series of chemical changes in your body. For instance, your endocrine system releases a steady stream of adrenaline, noradrenaline, and cortisol. When our bodies are undergoing stress, we take shallow, quick breaths, and we tense our shoulders. Excessive and long-term stress can have serious health implications, which I won't detail. Just know that our thoughts are serious business.

We have much more control over our thoughts than you might think. In fact, we have a phenomenal ability to manage our minds with just a little practice and self-awareness. One way you can change your life for the better, right now, is to gain control of your thoughts. The first step is to become aware. Simply observe your mind for a few days and see where it goes. When do you find your thoughts veering in a negative direction? Is it after a long day, when your husband comes home and doesn't give you the attention or love you are craving? Is it when your baby or toddler is needy and cranky? Do you find your thoughts becoming increasingly negative when you are hungry or tired, or in the presence of certain people?

Try to identify the individuals or events that trigger a series of negative thoughts for you. Then be more aware during these situations, to gain control over them. If you recognize that over-exhaustion and hunger trigger your negative thinking, for instance, do what you can to minimize these conditions. Exhaustion can be tough to avoid, but at least if you are aware of your tendencies, you can distract yourself with more positive circumstances when you are overly tired. And if hunger causes trouble for you, when you feel the pangs of hunger, eat!

There are also ways you can train your brain to be more efficient and organized. It sounds crazy, but once you calm the mental chatter, the remaining thoughts are much more intelligent, interesting, and useful. The best way to really clear your mind is to slow down and have times of quiet throughout the day. As I have said, meditation is the best tool out there to get to a place where your thoughts are as collected as possible. You might find your brain jumping all over at first ("monkey mind," as my yoga teacher calls it), but with time and practice, you can clear your mind and slow your pulse, and a new sense of inner peace will infuse your life.

Organize Your Closets

There is nothing better than waking up in the morning and having things run smoothly. If you work outside the home and have to take your baby to daycare, or have older children who have to get out the door to school, you know that a smooth morning is much harder to achieve when there are more of you to get up, dressed, fed, and out the door. One way you can make this easier on yourself is by organizing your closets. Why? Because when things are orderly, you can easily grab an outfit that fits and flatters you.

By this time, you have likely lost quite a few of your baby pounds and might feel ready to remove every last bit of maternity clothing from your closet. Whew! It feels so liberating to get rid of the bigger clothes! To begin, go through every item in your closet (you can do this very quickly), pulling out everything that is too big. Decide if you even want to keep it. Get a bag for the things you wish to donate, as well as a storage bin to hold your maternity clothes until the next time you need them. Or as is often the case, you might need to package them up and send them off to a sister or friend. Once you have gotten all of those clothes out of the way, organize everything that's left. I like to hang all of my jeans together, and my nice pants together; then I organize my shirts by color and style. I always fold my sweaters and put them on a shelf in my closet. Also, a nice rack can help you arrange your shoes nicely.

If you live in a seasonal climate, make sure your closet contains only the items for the season at hand; store the other things elsewhere if you can. Just think of anything you can do to make it easier to put together a cute outfit as quickly as possible.

Note the following characteristics of a well-organized closet:

— *It contains clothes that fit you well.* You shouldn't have to be discouraged by trying on three pairs of pants that are too tight. After having a baby, it might take some time to get to the size you want. Many of my friends have ended up buying jeans in a range of sizes. For example, if you are normally a size 6 (or strive to be), you might need a few pairs of size 8 and size 10 jeans in your closet for a while. The beautiful thing is that as you go through this book and slowly lose weight, you can put the bigger jeans away until you need them during your next pregnancy. If you become pregnant again, you can wear the bigger jeans in lieu of maternity jeans up to a certain point. My third pregnancy was a "whoops," and I had given away all of my maternity clothes. However, I had kept all of my bigger jeans, which got me by until my third trimester, when I finally broke down and bought a few pairs of maternity jeans.

— *It's full of clothes that you like and feel pretty in.* You shouldn't hang on to anything that you don't wear and don't really feel attractive in. Get rid of the clothes you don't love or can't see a good reason for keeping. Give them to someone who will enjoy them, making room for clothes that you adore and make you feel pretty.

— *It has good visibility.* You should be able to easily scan your closet and quickly find what you are looking for, or readily put together a great outfit.

— *It has easy accessibility.* Your life will run more smoothly if it's no trouble to grab any of the clothes from your closet without things falling out and making a big mess.

Organize Your Kitchen

I selected closets and kitchens as high-priority places to organize because I believe that when these places are orderly, the rest of our lives run just a bit more smoothly.

My mom recently watched my children so I could travel on a work trip. When I returned, I discovered that she had completely organized my pantry. It was beautiful! I felt compelled to maintain her order, and I am telling you, it is so much easier to find what I am looking for than it used to be. In fact, I felt inspired to arrange my other cupboards. I realized that even though it takes some time and effort to organize these places, it makes my daily life easier, and it's absolutely worth it.

Here are a few ideas for you:

— Once a week, before you or your partner goes to the grocery store, clean out your refrigerator. Scan for perishable items that have gone bad, and organize the shelves so similar items are grouped together. It also helps to put produce in the drawer that controls moisture and temperature, if your refrigerator has one. Your produce will last longer! With a paper towel, wipe down the shelves, including under the food, to keep the interior of your refrigerator nice and clean.

— If you have fruit or vegetables that you would eat more often if they were cut up, take the time to cut them up and put them in clear glass containers with sealable lids. That way you can stack them and see what's in there! You will be more likely to have these items as a healthy snack if they're easy to see and grab.

— Go through your storage containers, and get rid of random lids and containers that have no partner! I recommend using glass containers that have tight-fitting lids or plastic containers free of Bisphenol A (BPA) so that you don't have to worry about potentially harmful chemicals leaching into your food. Store each container with its lid so you don't have to search for it.

— Organize your pantry in a way that makes sense to you. For example, put all of your baking items together so it's easy to find exactly what you need when you decide to make some brownies. Keep a shelf full of healthy snacks for both you and your children. I also put all the breakfast items on a separate shelf. Do whatever it takes to be able to easily grab exactly what you need without a lot of searching.

In summary, organize the places in your home you use the most to help your life run more smoothly. Sometimes I need to reorganize my bath and beauty products when the area starts feeling a little chaotic, and the desk can get pretty messy when both my husband and I have our papers spread all over. This is not about being a neat freak; rather, I want to help you feel a sense of inner peace and ease throughout your day. Little complications like not being able to find a decent outfit to wear or clamoring to get breakfast ready can quickly compromise your mood! I believe firmly that we need to do everything we can to set ourselves up for happiness and ease in our daily lives.

Relinquishing Control

Let's face it: Many of us can be control freaks from time to time. We like to be able to direct our paths and have absolute power over the events and details of our day. At some point, we have to start letting go. Being a control freak can add stress and anxiety to your life at any time but even more so when you have babies. Motherhood can actually be one of life's funny lessons on letting go. As a mom, you will be late more often because of unforeseen events, such as diaper blowouts or spit-up messes, which require a trip back into the house for a wardrobe change. Our children are our greatest teachers to show us how to go with the flow and simply do the best we can.

Finding the right balance of keeping life peaceful while avoiding constant cleaning and fussing can be tough, but there is a time for everything. Clean when it's time to clean, and pick up a little throughout the day—but do not let this become obsessive.

While raising children, we have to learn to let our standards slide a bit and release control so we can fully enjoy our lives and experience the pleasures of motherhood.

Nourishment: Calories

Calorie—what a "weighty" word, with so much meaning for many of us. A calorie is just a measurement, but it has become tightly associated with deprivation, weight, and body image. *Calorie* is simply a technical word used to describe the amount of energy, or heat, required to raise the temperature of one kilogram of water one degree Celsius. In other words, calories measure the energy content, or the potential energy, of food.

We all need to eat enough calories to survive, and each of us has a basal metabolic rate (BMR) that dictates how many calories we need to be healthy. Each of us has a unique BMR based on our age, genetics, and other things that impact metabolism. If you are interested in figuring out how many calories you should be eating in general, here are the basic calculations. Keep in mind that this formula does not consider any factors other than gender, weight, height, age, and activity level. I do not suggest counting calories as a way of life at all, but I believe it is helpful to understand how much food your body really needs. At some point, I hope you are in touch with your body enough to feel how much you need to eat; but for me, after consuming larger quantities while being pregnant and nursing, I found it useful to count calories for just a few days to reset my normal inner eating gauge.

Step 1: Calculate Your BMR

Here is the formula for calculating BMR for women:

BMR = 655 + (4.3 × weight in pounds) + (4.7 × height in inches) − (4.7 × age in years)

I will do this calculation for myself, using my ideal weight:

*Erin's BMR (to maintain her ideal weight of 125 pounds) = 655 + (4.3 × 125) + (4.7 × 66.5) − (4.7 × 35) = **1,341 calories***

Note that this formula does not take into consideration nursing mothers. Mothers who nurse need an additional 300 to 600 calories each day, depending on the woman and the nutritional needs of the baby at the time. If a mother does not consume enough calories, her milk production may suffer, and she can quickly become malnourished. On a positive note, nursing a baby can burn as many calories as a five-mile run each day—which is just one of many reasons to nurse as long as you can.

Step 2: Calculate Your Activity

Now . . . here is the fun part. I enjoy this calculation because it helps you understand how important exercising is for achieving and maintaining a healthy weight. Simply put, physical activity speeds up your metabolism so that it burns calories more quickly. It is also a proven fact that muscle requires more calories than fat. Therefore, your body burns more calories, even while resting, when you have a higher percentage of muscle.

Remember that your BMR indicates the calories you need to eat just to live and perform basic bodily functions. You also need to determine the additional calories your body requires, based on your activity level.

- *If you are mostly sedentary (i.e., do very little exercise):* Multiply your BMR by 1.2. In my example, you would add 268 calories, for a total of 1,609 calories. Theoretically, this would be the number of calories that I could eat per day and maintain a weight of 125 if I did not exercise very often.

- *If you are lightly active (i.e., walk or do yoga one to three times a week)*: Multiply your BMR by 1.375. (My total would be 1,844 calories.)

- *If you are moderately active (i.e., do moderate exercise three to four days a week):* Multiply your BMR by 1.55. (My total would be 2,079 calories.)

- *If you are very active (i.e., run and do active sports for an hour a day, six to seven days a week):* Multiply your BMR by 1.725. (My total would be 2,313 calories.)

I am really hoping to highlight the major impact that exercising has on the amount of food you can eat. If you are a disciplined person and really want to get into the habit of eating enough calories to sustain your health *and* lose pounds, you can go write down everything you eat and then add up the calories. You can also calculate the calories you burn doing specific activities (such as aerobics, jogging, and even ironing!) using various calculators that are available. The best calorie-burning calculators take your weight into consideration, such as the one at **www.healthstatus .com/calculate/cbc.**

If you weigh 150 pounds but want to weigh 125, calculate your BMR as though you were a 125-pound woman. Then eat the quantity of food required to sustain the lower weight. Eventually, you should weigh 125 pounds. Additionally, by writing down your ideal weight in a place where you will see it frequently, you are basically letting the universe and your subconscious know what you should weigh. Then you can start visualizing and feeling yourself at that weight.

If you eat nourishing, healthy food and exercise regularly, *there should never be a need to count calories as a way of life.* Counting calories, in my opinion, takes the enjoyment out of eating and doesn't encourage us to get in touch with our bodies and simply eat good, nutritious food. In the beginning, it may be helpful to count calories so you can train yourself to feel how much food is the right amount. If you eat slowly and with awareness, your body will generally let you know when you have had enough. When you exercise, your appetite will be heartier, as it should be! For example, when you have a lazy day lounging around the house, you should find yourself getting too full if you eat the same quantity you did yesterday after a four-mile run.

I had to adjust the quantity of food I ate each time I stopped nursing. I remember I had been enjoying a slow but steady weight loss without trying too hard after each of my pregnancies, but I was working out most days and was nursing. Then . . . each time I weaned my babies, I found the scale stuck at a weight about five to ten pounds over where I wanted to be. After a few weeks of this,

I thought about the situation and realized I had become accustomed to eating an additional 300 to 500 calories each day, which I was easily burning off by nursing. Now that I wasn't nursing, my body didn't naturally require those additional calories. If I wanted to lose those last pounds, I was either going to have to exercise an additional 30 minutes to an hour each day or just eat a little less. Cutting 300 to 500 calories turned out to be pretty easy and resulted in my eliminating my nightly dessert (most of the time) and being a little more mindful of my portion sizes.

Many of my friends go through similar experiences after having babies. They are slowly but surely losing pounds; then one day, the scale just seems to stop moving south. This is an especially prevalent complaint in the 30-plus club. If this happens to you, it's time to reevaluate your habits and whether you are really eating well and getting enough sleep and exercise.

Check Your Progress
(Sleep + Exercise + Eating Well +
Body Love = Weight Loss)

This is a good time to evaluate how you are progressing toward your weight-loss goal. Is your weight going down, even if by just a few pounds? If the scale isn't moving, or not as quickly as you'd like, take this time to honestly evaluate how you are doing in the four key areas for weight loss success: adequate sleep, exercise, eating well, and body love.

Sleep

What can you be doing to make sure you are getting enough rest? I know I sometimes complain of being tired, but then I stay up late watching recorded episodes of *Modern Family* with my husband or reading an engrossing book. Love yourself enough to have the self-discipline to go to bed when you need to. No matter how much you believe that you don't need much sleep, research overwhelmingly proves that you do need adequate sleep to live at an optimal level. I want so see you thriving, feeling amazing, and bursting with energy.

Exercise

Are you making exercise an important part of your life? It can be tough to transition to incorporating physical fitness into your day, especially when just managing your life and caring for your baby can feel so overwhelming in and of themselves. Include exercise in your everyday life, and consider it as important as housekeeping and other daily tasks. Your health needs to be a priority so you can give your best to your family. The more you exercise, the better you will feel.

Eating Well

What have you been putting in your mouth? I discussed counting calories in great detail, but the ultimate goal is to get you to really know yourself and eat in a way that makes you feel great and optimizes your health. When you are truly in touch with your body, you will eat more of the things you know will make you feel good. Additionally, you will have a better idea of how much you need to eat to feel satisfied but not overly full. One thing I know about myself is that at restaurants, I have a compelling desire to eat everything on my plate. I am not usually a big fan of leftovers, and I don't like throwing away food. This knowledge helps me to share a meal or just order a smaller meal so I can clear my plate without feeling grossly overstuffed.

Body Love

How do you truly feel about your body? Do you need to retrain your habitual thought patterns? It can take a lot of practice to look at yourself in the mirror and truly love yourself, despite the imperfections you might see. Louise Hay, one of the foremost experts and authors related to personal growth, focuses a lot of her time and effort on getting people to do "mirror work." This essentially involves looking at yourself in the mirror and saying loving things. She starts with, "I love you." This can be a hard thing to say without laughing, but when the mother of self-help describes how she has assisted thousands of people to change their lives for the better with this small practice, I take it seriously. It's even harder to do while naked. It might take as long as a month to do it with a straight face, but give it a try. When you truly love yourself and accept your body, I promise that taking care of yourself and making the lifestyle changes necessary to reach your body's ideal weight will be infinitely easier.

Fitness: Making Exercise Part of Your Daily Routine

Over time, your workouts will simply become part of your life. Then, when you don't exercise for a few days, you will start to feel a little off and actually miss your workouts! It is my hope that after three months of following the schedules and suggestions in this book, you will actually enjoy your workouts and appreciate how great you feel afterward—so much so that they become part of your daily routine.

One thing moms need to be is efficient with their time. Longer, slower workouts can be wonderful to burn calories and build stamina, but research shows that intense, quick workouts are an important piece for getting in shape and toning your muscles. I have seen multiple women get in the best shape of their lives doing CrossFit workouts, which take between 20 and 30 minutes, plus a warm-up. Granted, these workouts are really tough, and it takes a while to be able to do them exactly as prescribed. But if you are interested in taking your workouts to a new level, check out CrossFit's workout of the day (**www.crossfit.com**); then do it at home or at a local gym. Otherwise, there are dozens of fabulous and intense workout videos that can be done in 20 to 45 minutes. Just remember, the shorter your workouts, the more you need to push up the intensity to make it worthwhile!

This week's workout schedule, below, is intended to encourage you to keep moving forward and help you set the goal of fitting in each of the workouts listed. You are doing great!

Week 5 Workout Schedule

Monday	Tuesday	Wednesday	Thursday	Friday	Saturday	Sunday
30-minute walk or 20-minute jog	20 minutes strength	1-hour walk, 30-minute jog, or cardio class at gym	20 minutes strength	30-minute walk, 20-minute jog, or cardio class at gym	Yoga or Pilates class	Rest

Awesome Arm Workout

I remember seeing a photo of myself at one of my baby showers in a sleeveless dress while eight months pregnant. I was appalled at how my arms looked, especially with the way I was posing (with my arms pressed to my sides). I love the look of toned arms and wanted them dearly after giving birth. Moms need to have strong arms so they can carry the heavy objects that having a baby requires, such as infant car seats. Before doing this workout, do some jumping jacks to get blood pumping throughout your body. Be sure to have some five-, eight-, or ten-pound dumbbells on hand.

1. *Bicep Curls.* Holding five- to ten-pound dumbbell weights, allow your arms to hang naturally by your sides, with the dumbbells turned inward. Twist your wrists so that your palms face up, and lift both dumbbells straight up to your shoulders. Slowly release your bicep back down to the starting position. Repeat 10 to 20 times.

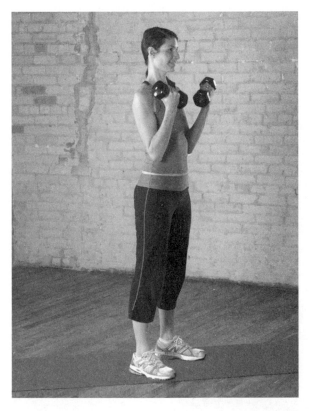

2. *Alternating Cross-Chest Bicep Curls.* Holding five- to ten-pound dumbbell weights, allow your arms to hang naturally by your sides, with the dumbbells turned inward. Starting with your right arm, twist your wrist so that your palm faces up, and lift the weight slowly to the left shoulder. Slowly release your bicep back down to the starting position, and then switch by bringing your left hand to your right shoulder. Repeat 10 to 20 times on each side.

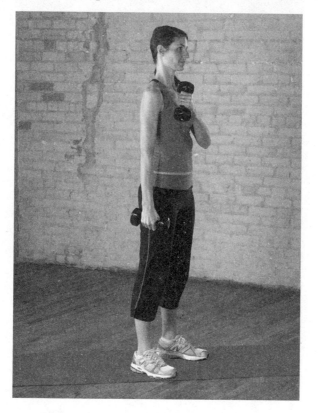

3. *Dips.* Start by sitting on a chair or bench. Place the palms of your hands on the edge of your chair. Keeping your knees bent at a 90-degree angle or straight out, lift your body off and down until your elbows are bent to a 90-degree angle. Slowly push back up until your arms are straight, and repeat 10 to 15 times.

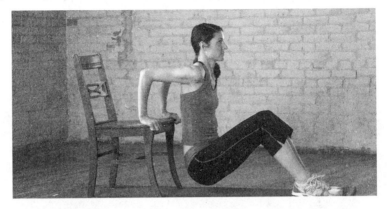

4. *Shoulder Flies.* Grasp five- or eight-pound dumbbells in front of your thighs, with your elbows and knees both slightly bent. Bend over slightly and raise your arms straight out to your sides until your elbows are shoulder height. Lower and repeat 10 to 15 times.

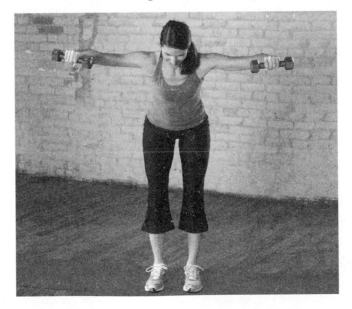

5. *Push-ups.* Start in the plank/push-up position, with your hands slightly more than shoulder-width apart. You can perform these on either your toes or your knees, but keep your body straight. Lower your body by bending your elbows, until you are an inch or two from the ground. Repeat 10 to 15 times.

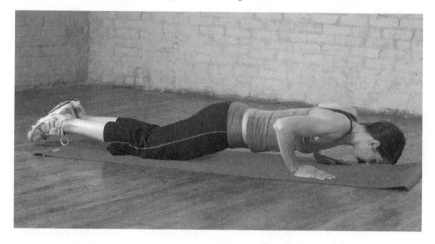

Sanity Saver: Social Outlets

Being home with a new baby can be extremely fulfilling but at the same time isolating. Many moms I know complain of loneliness and boredom. I generally find my time at home with my kids to be busy and enjoyable, but after a few days of just hanging around the house, I start feeling a little stir-crazy and in desperate need of adult interaction! After the six-week go-ahead from my doctor after giving birth, I started going to the gym as much for the social interaction as for the exercise. It was fun to show off my new baby and start working on getting my body to start resembling its original shape and size.

I feel the need for social interaction more acutely when my husband is working long hours or is out of town. Sometimes I just have to make sure that I have fun things scheduled both with and without my kids. I love getting up in the morning and jogging with the stroller, going to the local coffee shop to pick up a latte, and walking home. I bribe my older daughter to stay in the stroller with chocolate milk. Yes, before becoming a mom, I had said I would never bribe my kids, but it is so darn effective that I now call it "positive reinforcement." I am all for it, if it allows me to sit at a coffee shop and enjoy a latte and the newspaper or a magazine for 15 minutes. This is also a chance to chat with the friendly barista, who knows just how I like my coffee; and I always run into a person or two that I know.

My friends and I also highly recommend arranging play dates. Play dates can be wonderful, but they can also be a little stressful if you're not careful. I had a really awesome friend, who has two children, over the other day. My friend's toddler is a gorgeous little terror who kept poking my little ones, screaming, climbing up on the table, and pulling things down, making for a non-relaxing atmosphere. The older kids hardly played; instead, they fought over toys. After cleaning my house all morning to have guests over, the place was trashed and I was exhausted. I have also been the one at other people's houses with a toddler who acts like a tornado and makes a huge mess, so I know how nerve-racking that feels, too.

Overall, play dates are usually fun and rewarding for both moms and children. The point is to have people over whom you enjoy and who won't cause you more stress than enjoyment.

A lot of moms use social media sites, such as Facebook, for social interaction. As a military spouse, I use Facebook like crazy to keep up with friends from all the stages of my life and places we've lived. It's a great way to keep in touch, but it's no substitute for face-to-face human interaction.

Don't forget about getting dressed up and going out, both with your girlfriends and with your partner. When my second baby was 12 weeks old and my husband was deployed, I got a babysitter for a few hours, squeezed my rear into some cute jeans, fixed my hair, put on makeup, wore sassy shoes, and met up with some girlfriends for a glass of wine. I came home much more relaxed, happy, and "myself" again after some fun and adult conversation.

A supportive and empathetic circle of girlfriends is a must for any mom. Getting out with women who will listen to your complaints and concerns, understand your troubles and stresses, and celebrate your successes is as critical to your well-being as eating well and exercising. It can be hard to nurture these relationships when your life is so busy and consumed with raising children, but at this time, these relationships are more important than ever.

Is your partner willing to stay home with the children to allow you a night away? Maybe you can both plan nights out with your friends and get a babysitter. Both women and men need the support of same-sex friends because, quite frankly, we aren't able to support our men in ways that other men can, and men generally can't support us in the same way our girlfriends can. It's a basic difference between the sexes. I know there are exceptions to this, but an extraordinary life will include great relationships with a partner and with a nurturing, fun group of friends.

Plan a girls' night out. Look in the paper for an upcoming concert that you know there's no way your man would want to attend, or a chick flick that you'd have to drag him to. Sometimes meeting for dinner or drinks is the most fun because it allows you time to just catch up and talk. There is something so therapeutic about these conversations, often languishing over delicious meals or fun, girly drinks. Even an afternoon excursion for a late lunch, shopping, or coffee can do the trick if evenings are tough.

Get dressed up in something vivacious and fun—something you feel really cute in. Sometimes it's entertaining to text with your girlfriends while getting ready to see what they are wearing—just like you did in high school (although you might have had to pick up the phone back then). It might seem juvenile, but it's just plain fun! Your girlfriends will appreciate your fashionable ensemble more than your husband, and I think sharing an interest in clothing is just one of the ways that women bond.

Affirmation for the Week

Feeling organized and in control is a crucial and often underempha-sized part of inner peace. Beautiful and uncluttered surroundings allow my brain to have more focus and release creative energy. I will arrange my life so that it simply flows. Stressful moments of clamoring to find things or rushing to get ready in the morning will be minimized, as a more Zen feeling takes over in my home.

★☐★

Reviving Relationships

"A loving relationship is one in which the loved one is free to be himself—to laugh with me, but never at me; to cry with me, but never because of me; to love life, to love himself, to love being loved. Such a relationship is based upon freedom and can never grow in a jealous heart."

—LEO F. BUSCAGLIA

While babies can help partners bond, they can also be tremendously hard on romantic relationships. A marriage can collapse due to the strain of raising children and the lack of energy put into the relationship. A study performed at the University of Washington found that 67 percent of married couples reported that their marital satisfaction had dropped significantly since their first child was born. Additionally, the average couple underwent eight times more marital conflict after having children.[1]

The primary reasons for the dramatic increase in marital discomfort are the substantial drop in time spent connecting with each other, as well as a dramatic decrease in personal time for rest and rejuvenation. How can you have anything left for your spouse when you haven't taken the time to care for yourself? Children's needs are imperative and often must be met immediately, while tending to your partner's needs often feels optional—saved for the rare occasion when time and energy allow. This depressing and gloomy trend can be turned around, if you take the time to care for yourself so you have something left for your spouse.

Friendships change. It's tough to make time with friends a priority when schedules are already constrained. Women depend on their connections with other women for nurturing and emotional support. When things get really tough in life, it's generally your girlfriends who love and support you in that uniquely loving and encouraging way. It is ideal to have both a loving relationship with your husband and a thick network of empathetic girlfriends.

In particular, many moms notice changes in their relationships with girlfriends who don't have children. I will never forget a visit from a kid-free friend while my husband was out of town. At the time, we were living in a gorgeous beach community, and my friend had planned for us to spend our days at the water and our evenings at the clubs. I told her I would line up babysitters, but in my mind, one or two nights out would have been fantastic. We had a fundamental difference in expectations, which ended in disaster. She arrived and showed her continual disappointment through frowns, sighs, and complaints. Each of us left the visit with hard feelings toward each other. We have since talked about what happened, worked it out, and completely moved on, with the understanding that we are simply on different life paths right now; but I don't want any of you to have to go through these struggles.

Even relationships within the larger family can change and become challenging after a child arrives. Women need connections with their relatives to be strong and supportive at a time when it's tough to nourish these key relationships.

This week, I will offer numerous suggestions for women to get their relationships back on track.

Your Relationship with Your Husband or Partner

There are few things that have the ability to rock a marriage like starting a family. While having a baby is one of the most special and intimate things you can ever do with another human being, it also has the great potential to drive a substantial wedge between the two of you. You might be so busy and tired that you haven't had the energy to notice—which is half the trouble.

When my second child was a newborn, I was living in an exhausted, lonely blur. My husband had gone to Hawaii for many weeks on a military assignment. I could feel a wedge of disconnection between us, but I had no idea how far our relationship had deteriorated. Between his absence over 50 percent of the time for military work and our two young children, there was animosity and distance on both sides of our relationship. Things came to a terrible head, and we were forced to face our problems and finally communicate. Thankfully, our deep love and desire to keep our family together prompted us to reexamine our lives and make some dramatic changes. I could see numerous places where we'd both gone wrong. I'd like to help other women learn from my mistakes, which I see women in my life making with their spouses every day.

From the father's perspective, you have been taken over by this child. Someone other than him has hijacked your body, your mind, your energy, and most of your time. It is very easy for Mom to become singularly focused on the baby while Dad is left on the sidelines wondering if he will ever get you back. I didn't realize this the first time I went through it, and not until a while after the second baby was born did I understand how my behavior was alienating my husband. He was lonely and felt very out of touch with me, but I was too wrapped up to notice. I also held a bit of resentment because I felt as though I had to do all the work for the baby and for keeping up our home. By the third baby, things went beautifully because I was aware of how my husband felt, and we were able to communicate and do things to make our relationship a priority as much as possible.

Here are some of the key challenges that can arise for couples with new babies:

- Mom's body has undergone some substantial changes, making her feel self-conscious and unsexy.

- Mom's breasts are engorged and leaking milk, making her feel more like a heifer than a Hugh Hefner girl.

- Mom is often the primary baby feeder, so she is up at all hours of the night getting more and more exhausted

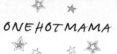

and worn down, to the point where sex feels like one of the last things in the world she wants to do.

- Dad understands that his woman is exhausted, but he feels helpless and as though he doesn't have a lot to offer early on.

- Men are problem solvers, and when they can't solve a problem (like a baby who won't stop screaming), they feel very frustrated.

- Dad is intimidated and a little leery of Mom's body and all it has gone through.

- Dad just wants to have an intelligent conversation with his wife that doesn't involve the baby's bowels or latest skills.

- Dad wants someone to listen to him and pay attention to his needs but feels guilty for wanting more from his wife because he can see that she's spent.

There are many more, but you get the picture. You and your partner are likely experiencing this baby thing in two very different ways. The best way to find out what's going on with your partner is to sit down and talk. You need to set aside time to just be together and catch up, which leads me to one of my first suggestions.

Take Time to Reconnect

When was the last time you and your partner sat down at the end of the day and sipped leisurely on a glass of wine while bringing each other up to date on your lives? Better yet, when was the last time you had an engaging discussion about politics or your dreams together? If you are like the majority of couples with young children, you might say it's been a while.

Successful couples generally do the following: communicate openly, resolve to work through problems and conflict, make each other their number one priority, and schedule time together alone. You heard me. *You need to put your spouse before the baby.* This doesn't mean that you ignore your hungry or screaming child. It means that your marriage is the central relationship in your family. Happy marriages equal happy children.

An article in *Scientific American Mind* discussing the most important "parenting competencies" listed "love and affection" and "relationship skills" as two of the most important things that influence a child's health, happiness, and success in school.[2] This article was referring to a healthy and loving relationship between the parents, which models effective relationship skills for children. In addition, it makes children feel secure.

You need to make time to nurture your romantic relationship. Give it the attention it needs wherever and whenever you can. Now that you have a baby, you might not be able to just fit it in; you will probably also have to schedule it in. Find someone you trust to watch the baby, even if it's just for an hour or two at first, so you and your husband can get out and reconnect over dinner or a hike.

We will discuss ways to reignite your sexual relationship later. Before you can even get there, you need to be sure you are connected emotionally and mentally first. Women, in particular, need this connection before they are ready to really enjoy the physical stuff. How can you reconnect with your partner? Here are a few ideas for you to consider implementing into your life. These suggestions were offered by dozens of women involved in happy marriages while raising babies and children:

— Touch each other a lot, and kiss each time you return home to each other.

— Be on his team (more on this below).

— Talk on the phone or text at least once a day. This might seem corny, but I know a lot of husbands really like it. If your husband is not a real phone person or is not able to talk at work, a quick text to say hello works great.

— Schedule a date night once a week, even if it's a "state" (what my husband and I call a night together at home spent hanging out, watching a movie, enjoying a game of cards, or having a drink together after the kids go to bed).

— Take a moment to greet each other at the end of the day and catch up. The book *On Becoming Baby Wise* recommends that parents have "couch time" at the end of the day. This involves entertaining your children otherwise, sitting on the couch, and simply focusing on each other for 15 minutes. We can do this occasionally, but generally my husband comes home pretty late and we end up chatting while finishing dinner. The point is to be genuinely interested in each other's day and how things went.

The simple act of staying connected and keeping the lines of communication wide open will do amazing things for your relationship. Be in touch enough to realize when something feels off, such as your partner is acting a little distant. Ask him if everything's okay in a way that is friendly. If something is really bothering you, bring it up. Don't raise too many issues at once, but if something bugs you for more than a week, it needs to be discussed. Otherwise, you might start taking it out on him, even if it's completely subconscious.

Another thing that will keep you connected with your husband is showing an interest in what he's doing. Be involved and ask questions. For example, my husband loves when I can engage in a discussion about the type of flight he did at work that day. He feels like we are a real team when I attend his work functions and know about what is going on at work. Be interested in his friends and treat them well.

Men like to feel that their wives are "on their team." We women also like to feel that our men have our backs. As a Pollyanna type of person, I try to see the best in people. So in the past, when my husband would come home from work and vent or complain about someone, my typical response would be something like, "I am sure he's actually a great guy and didn't mean it like that" or

"He must have just been having a bad day." In my mind, I was helping my husband see humanity in a brighter light. To Steve, I was telling him that his feelings were invalid and I was downplaying how he felt. Instead of being his best friend, I was "siding with the enemy" from his viewpoint. He would often say, "Hey, be on my team." Steve is definitely my best friend in many respects, but sometimes I take him for granted and don't spend time giving him what he needs from a friendship standpoint. What he needs is someone who is going to be on his side and whom he can count on to listen and be empathetic when he has crappy days. Isn't that really what we all want?

So remember to pay attention to your partner's subtle cues that you are or aren't giving him what he needs. Be his friend, and be on his side. It's a long haul through life together, and it will be so much more fun if you are on the same team.

Communicate

This goes hand in hand with reconnecting, but it's so important that I am going to give it a little more coverage. Communicate every day, about every little thing, both good and bad. Tell him about your day, and be interested in hearing about his. Let him know about the little things that are bothering you so he doesn't have to play a guessing game. Men like things to be straightforward. They don't like trying to figure things out based on our moods. As clear as things may seem to you, I can almost guarantee you that it isn't that clear to him.

Your relationship with your husband can start to feel very distant and lonely when you aren't talking to each other. I know this from experience. There are many weeks in my marriage when my husband and I feel so busy that we don't connect and hardly talk. At times I have been a little cranky for reasons that make perfect sense to me: I am completely exhausted from taking care of our entire house; caring for the kids and all of our appointments, gifts, grocery shopping, meals, etc.; and working and writing a book on top of it. Yet he doesn't ask what's wrong; he just assumes he has pissed me off and gives me some space. Can't he see why I am cranky? Surprisingly, he can't. He just thinks I am being bitchy, takes it personally, and avoids deep discussions because he's wondering what he did wrong. Does this sound familiar?

When Steve and I finally sit down and spend some time together, I tell him how overworked and completely spent I feel. He is not only empathetic but also asks how he can help more. We then discuss having a housekeeper come every few weeks to help with the deep cleaning. Whew! Exactly what I need. From my standpoint, the source of my exhaustion is perfectly obvious. But I can't stress this enough: Men don't always get it. Most of us didn't marry jerks; we married human beings who often see the world quite differently than we do.

Communicate Effectively

When we reconnect regularly, we communicate more often. This is a great start. Another key to communication is speaking in a way that your partner will hear. Effective communication is key for all areas of life but in particular between spouses. My friends and I have discussed the following pattern: We try to let little things go and don't bring them up until they build up more and more until we nearly explode. At that point, we communicate with anger and frustration. We instantly put our partners on the defense. I know that when I've gotten to that point, my husband doesn't really listen to what I am saying; he just puts up his defenses. Using certain words and phrases can be immediately inflammatory. Here are some ways of starting sentences that do not usually elicit the responses we are hoping for:

- "You always . . ."
- "What's wrong with you?" and other insulting phrases
- "Why can't you . . . ?"

When your partner responds to whatever it is you have to say, take a deep breath and become completely present before you fire back any kind of reply. Emotional responses will not always convey what we really feel and intend. What you want to do is disarm your partner so you can have a rational, adult conversation that accomplishes something and moves your relationship forward. Do not have an emotional or heated discussion when you are already exhausted or not in a good place, because you may not have enough control over your reactions.

Be Direct

I can't stress this enough. When your man asks you a question, give him a straight answer to the question he asked. When polling men about how women can communicate better with them, nearly all of them said they wanted women to be clear and concise. Here is a hilarious example that was given by a friend's husband: "Answer the question that I asked, not what you think I wanted to hear or an explanation of events. For example: *Question*: Would you like me to pick us up some dinner? *Bad answer #1*: Oh, I don't know, what do you want to do? *Bad Answer #2*: Well, I don't want you to have to go out of your way. I know you've had a busy day, so maybe I can just make something or . . . maybe you could just stop somewhere easy. *Good Answer*: Yes, I'd love to have Chinese from XY Restaurant."

Women have a way of wanting to explain things. Instead of giving a clear answer, we often give all kinds of ancillary data, like our girlfriends would enjoy hearing. Our men truly just want us to be straightforward. I have to be very conscious to be successful with this one, but it's important if we want to be effective and get the results we want in life.

Make Your Partner Feel Special

One of the other best things you can do to baby-proof your marriage is to go out of your way to make your husband feel special. I know, he is the one who should be making *you* feel special since you're the one who delivered the baby and does most of the work, but I promise that (usually) the more you give, the more you get.

As I have mentioned, men can feel a little threatened by the baby, mostly because the baby takes you and the majority of your attention away from him. You need to make him feel extra special so he still knows how very important he is to you. Most men have much more fragile egos than they let on, so we need to stroke them from time to time. How can we do this? Here are a few ideas:

— In addition to texting hello, text him that he is hot in the middle of the day.

— Celebrate his successes in a big way. Did he just get a promotion? Then hire a babysitter, make a reservation at the nicest restaurant in town, and put on a sexy shirt. Even if he just passed a test or achieved some other milestone, make his favorite dinner or get him a special treat.

— Write each other notes. My husband often has to get up really early to go to work, so we have a pad of paper on the counter where we write each other little love notes. Some are even as simple as, "Have a great day!"

— Flirt with him. Other women probably do, so you should do it the most and be the very best at it.

— Bring him coffee or some type of treat at work (occasionally). I will never forget bringing our couple-week-old baby to Steve's squadron and watching him parade around the building showing off his daughter to his buddies with a look of pure pride. It was precious! I have also brought him a surprise lunch before, and I know it makes his day.

— Compliment him shamelessly. Tell him he looks great when he leaves for work. Notice when he gets his haircut, and be sure to let him know it looks good. When he fixes something in the house or does something for you, thank and praise him up and down.

— Applaud his fathering skills. Most men do not come to parenthood as easily as women do. They need to know they are doing an okay job, and any positive feedback will help. He will also want to help more if he is being praised for what he is already doing.

Your Relationships with Your Girlfriends

Study after study shows that the happiest people have trustworthy and supportive friends. Mothers, in particular, thrive with a network of healthy, compassionate, and encouraging friendships. Women need to learn how to attract the right people into their lives and spend time with those who bring them joy. Cultivating friendships can be learned, and women who take the time to nourish their relationships will be much more fulfilled in other areas of life.

Many new mothers have amazing girlfriends but don't feel that they have enough time or energy to nurture these relationships. As a mom, I have met some special new friends but didn't make a lot of effort to connect because I just didn't feel that I had the extra time.

Women who work outside the home in addition to having babies feel this even more acutely. One of my dear friends, Christine, works full-time as an executive. At the end of the day, she thinks of nothing other than getting home with her children to spend some time with them. She works out during her lunch hour, so she really has very little extra time to cultivate her relationships. What she has going for her is an extensive network of old friends whom she calls on her long drives to and from work and on weekends. She can let her guard down with these long-time confidantes. So while she isn't necessarily making new friends, she is doing what she must to keep her system of well-established relationships healthy and intact.

How can you sustain your friendships when you feel so busy?

— Keep a calendar marked with your friends' birthdays and special events. Maintain a drawer with numerous beautiful birthday cards so it's easy to get cards off in time to make your special women feel loved.

— Call your best friends when you have a long drive ahead of you, using a hands-free device, of course! Use one naptime per week to call or e-mail those friends who have been on your mind.

— E-mail photos of your baby for your friends to enjoy—not too many, but enough that they can feel part of your life and connected to your family's new addition.

— Send quick notes and e-mails to your closest friends regularly. This doesn't have to take long. Just let them know you are thinking about them and share what's going on in your life.

— I have mentioned this already, but get a babysitter or have your husband watch the kid(s) so you can enjoy a girls' night or afternoon out. You will actually be able to complete full conversations without interruption when the kids are elsewhere. You truly need these kid-free times to connect with your friends on a deeper level.

— That said, get together for coffee with your friends and bring the babies. If you wait until you are baby-free, you might not get to see each other very often. It's also great to have a reason to get up and dressed, go out, and have conversations that you just can't always have with your husband. Maybe you need to discuss something you are going through, and your girlfriends are the perfect sounding board.

Girlfriends Who Don't Have Children

This is a special and important group of friends to have. They will promptly return your e-mails and phone calls, will go for a crazy night out at a moment's notice, and will have interesting and wild stories to entertain you when you aren't doing much besides hanging out at home. Do not ignore these friendships or let them go by the wayside. These girls will help you keep things in perspective!

There are a few things to keep in mind, however. Women who don't have kids don't understand how difficult and crazy having children can be. Let them know you are busy, but don't complain constantly or make excuses. Some of these women get it, while others don't. They are going to be interested in your children but only to an extent. Use these women to stay true to who you are. They want to have deep and interesting conversations with you, like they always have. They are not interested in bonding over your cracked nipples or how much weight your baby has gained. They might feign interest for a while, but these women are the ones who just want you to be you.

It is important to set expectations with these women if they live out of town and come to stay at your home for a visit. They will expect you to be able to go out and do things, just like normal. You need to set expectations at the onset of the visit that you have a babysitter for one night, for example, but otherwise you hang out with her at home. Just communicate to make sure you both leave your time together feeling satisfied and happy.

Nourishment: The Real Skinny on Fat

Fat has gotten a really bad rap, and it's not entirely fair. There are certainly bad fats, but there are also many good fats that are essential for health. This section contains a little "fat primer" to help you understand fat and make better food choices—so you don't become, or remain, fat.

Not-So-Good Fats

There are a few types of fat that are particularly bad for your health, including trans fats and saturated fats. These two types of fat are known to have a negative impact on your blood cholesterol and can cause serious health problems over time if eaten in large quantities. Try to limit your intake of these not-so-good fats.

Trans Fat

Trans fat, also known as hydrogenated fat or partially hydrogenated oil, can be encountered in some meat and dairy products but is primarily found in processed foods. Most trans fats are manmade, created by adding hydrogen to unsaturated fats. This process makes a fat product, which is easier to cook with and gives products a longer shelf life. Problematically, these substances are not natural, and our bodies do not respond well to them. In fact, synthetic trans fats are linked to higher levels of LDL (low-density lipoprotein, also known as bad cholesterol) and lower levels of HDL (high-density lipoprotein, also known as good cholesterol), leading to a higher risk of cardiovascular disease. Trans fats can be found in baked goods, cookies, crackers, and other processed foods and should be avoided as much as possible.

Saturated Fat

Saturated fat comes primarily from animal sources and is known to raise blood cholesterol levels as well as LDL (bad) cholesterol levels. Excessive consumption of saturated fat is also linked to an increased risk of type 2 diabetes.

Much Better Fats

Monounsaturated and polyunsaturated fats (omega-3 and omega-6 fatty acids) are much better for you than trans fat and saturated fat. They generally come from natural food sources. Fat is still fat and should be eaten in moderation; however, some of these types of fats are actually essential for living your healthiest life and feeling fabulous. Read on!

Monounsaturated Fat

Monounsaturated fat, also known as monounsaturated fatty acid (MUFA), is healthier fat. It is liquid at room temperature. Monounsaturated fats are found naturally in foods like red meat; whole milk products; nuts; and high-fat fruits, such as olives and avocados. Other sources include grapeseed oil, peanut oil, sesame oil, popcorn, whole-grain wheat, oatmeal, safflower oil, and sunflower oil. This fat can be very good for you in moderation and usually contains antioxidants and nutrients such as vitamin E. Monounsaturated fats are also shown to lower the levels of LDL (bad) cholesterol in your blood, lower your risk of heart disease and stroke, and help maintain healthy cells.

Polyunsaturated Fat

Polyunsaturated fats are found in natural, whole foods such as nuts, fish, and leafy greens and include the essential fatty acids (EFAs): omega-3 and omega-6 fatty acids. There is also an omega-9 fatty acid; however, it is not considered an EFA because it can be created from unsaturated fat by the human body.

Omega-3 fatty acids, also known as polyunsaturated fatty acids (PUFAs), are found in most fish, such as salmon; other seafood, including algae and krill; some plants; and nut oils. Omega-3s are crucial for vibrant health, and their benefits include reducing the risk of heart disease, cancer, arthritis, and stroke—as well as decreasing symptoms of depression, hypertension, and attention deficit hyperactivity disorder (ADHD). Omega-3 fatty acids are crucial for healthy brain functioning. They also help control inflammation in our tissues, joints, and blood. Inflammation occurs when the body releases white blood cells and other inflammatory chemicals in an effort to protect itself from infection or a foreign substance (such as bacteria or a virus). Omega-3s can also prevent and/or minimize autoimmune disease, and are known to help improve health related to the following conditions:

- High cholesterol. (Omega-3s increase HDL—good cholesterol—and reduce triglycerides, which are fats in the blood.)

- High blood pressure

- Heart disease. (Eating at least two servings of fish per week can reduce the risk of stroke by as much as 50 percent.)

- Diabetes

- Rheumatoid arthritis

- Depression and bipolar disorder

- Cognitive decline

- Skin disorders

- Inflammatory bowel disease (IBD)

- Asthma

- Macular degeneration

- Menstrual pain

- Colon, breast, and prostate cancer

Omega-6 fatty acids are another category of fats. They are more commonly found in the typical American diet, in foods like poultry, eggs, cereal, margarine, and vegetable oil. Omega-6s are also essential to our health and promote healthy skin and cholesterol levels.

The problem that not many of us are aware of is that there is an ideal balance of omega-6 and omega-3 fatty acids in our diet. This is a *4:1 ratio,* or four parts omega-3s to one part omega-6s. The typical American diet tends to contain 14 to 25 times more omega-6 fatty acids than omega-3 fatty acids, which is a ratio that can promote clot formation in the blood and increase the risk of heart attack and stroke.[3]

Fitness: Why You Should Consider Group Fitness

Working out at a gym with others has numerous benefits. First of all, it provides an opportunity to get out of the house and potentially make some new friends. Second, if you go to a class, you will usually stick it out to the end and work out longer and harder than you might have on your own. Finally, you will get out of your comfort zone and work out your entire body. And there are so many classes that make it fun to burn calories.

Thankfully, there is a variety of classes to suit all fitness levels. For example, you might try a spinning class and keep the bike on an easier level until you are ready to push yourself harder. You can make any of these classes your own, taking it down a notch when needed or pushing yourself when you're up for it. Try Zumba, which is one of the most fun fitness classes I have done in a long time. Weight classes are super effective; just be sure to start at a level that is true to your current condition. Take it easy until you are ready!

Gyms are weatherproof and often offer childcare, so there are two more excuses that will no longer work if you join a gym! The workout schedule for Week 6 could be accomplished entirely at a gym, using cardio and weight equipment supplemented with a couple of challenging classes. Ideally, the schedule will help you determine ahead of time which workouts you want to do at home and which ones you'd rather do at a gym. Don't forget that all of these workouts can also be performed at home if that works better for you and your baby's schedule.

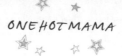

Week 6 Workout Schedule

Monday	Tuesday	Wednesday	Thursday	Friday	Saturday	Sunday
45-minute walk or 30-minute jog	20 minutes strength	1-hour walk, 30-minute jog, or cardio class at gym	20 minutes strength	30-minute walk, 20-minute jog, or cardio class at gym	Yoga or Pilates class	Rest

Pilates Power Workout

Pilates is one of the very best ways to strengthen and tone your body, and it's an ideal workout for new mothers. Pilates really targets your core muscles, which have a tendency to weaken through pregnancy and delivery. Try doing the following entire set of Pilates exercises three times through.

1. *The Hundred.* Lie with your back flat on the floor. Use your abs to raise both legs and your head a few inches off the floor, with your arms stretched out next to your sides. Be sure to keep your neck neutral and your chin tucked. Begin to lift and lower your arms from about two to ten inches from the floor, while inhaling on the lift and exhaling on the lower. Do this for five up-and-down beats, and repeat 10 times until you have reached 100.

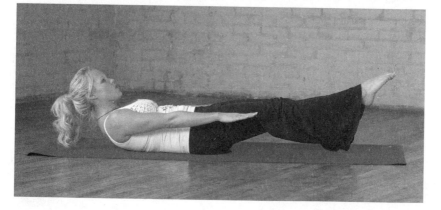

2. *Crisscross.* Start by lying on your back with your head and shoulders lifted off the floor, hands behind your head, and knees into your chest. Extend your left leg a few inches off of the floor, and then lift your right leg up and grab behind your right knee. Hold for three counts, and then switch sides. Be sure your abdominal muscles are engaged the entire time! Try to do this exercise ten times on each side.

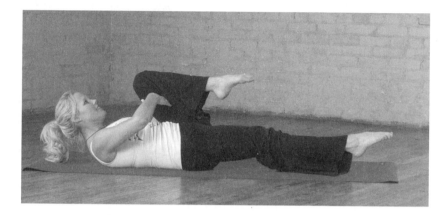

3. *Leg Circles.* Lie on your back with your hands supporting your neck. Use your abs to engage your core, and lift your head and shoulders slightly off the floor. Your right leg will be straight up. Circle your right toes in a two- to three-foot radius. Circle 10 times clockwise and then 10 times counterclockwise. Switch legs and repeat.

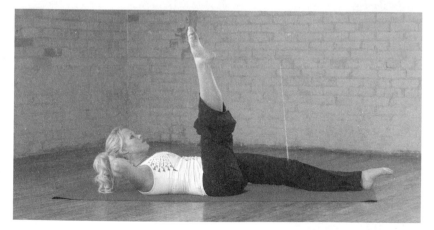

4. *Donkey Kickbacks*. Start by kneeling on the floor, keeping your spine neutral and your toes tucked under. Contract your abs as you bring your right knee to your nose, then kick that leg straight back behind you, squeezing your gluteus and keeping your abs tight. Repeat 10 times total and then repeat on the other side.

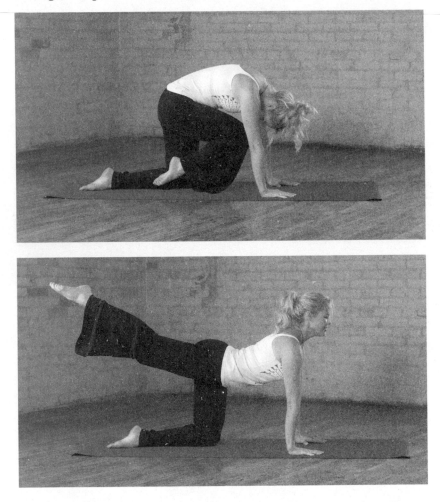

5. *The Roll-Up.* Lie on your back with your legs straight and your arms stretched above your head. Gradually lift your arms toward the ceiling as you inhale. As you exhale, slowly roll forward as you peel your spine off the floor. As you inhale again, stretch your body and arms out over your legs with your eyes focused forward. Finally, exhale and slowly roll all the way back down to the floor. Continue with the next repetition as you inhale, and complete 10 repetitions.

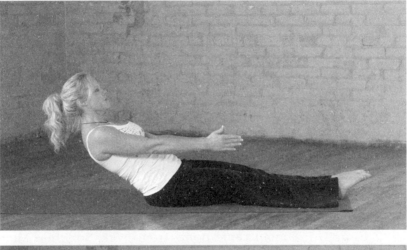

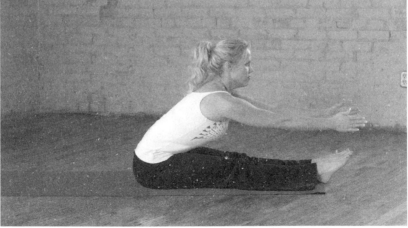

Sanity Saver: Developing a Support Network

These days, many of us are raising children far from our families and closest friends. As a military family, we are painfully aware that we don't have an extensive backup system when we move to a new place; it can feel very lonely. Military folks are incredible about supporting one another, but it can be hard to reach out and ask for help from people who are not family.

There is something so true about the African proverb, "It takes a village to raise a child." Raising children is such an important and demanding job that the more people you've got supporting you, the better. Moms of past generations were much more likely to live within a few minutes of their own mothers, sisters, and cousins. Family and lifelong friends spanned generations and sustained each other in countless ways. Women supported each other and offered parenting advice. Childcare wasn't as much of an issue because most women didn't work. When they wanted to go out on a date with their husbands, needed some personal time, or had an appointment, a dozen individuals were happy to help.

My own grandmother lived a few miles away while I grew up, and she met my brother and me every day after school and stayed with us until my mom came home from work. So while Mom worked full-time, it never really felt like a burden. My grandmother made everything fun, always welcoming us home with a hug and a cookie. I am sad to say that my own mom now lives three plane rides or a 24-hour drive away. There are many days when I ache to have someone around whom I can depend on and who loves my children as much as I do.

If we don't have family nearby, and sometimes even when we do, we need to create support networks. Raising children is a big job, and sometimes we simply need backup. I've had to create support networks in numerous new towns, and the stress level in my life drops greatly as soon as I do. There is nothing more nerve-racking than being in a pickle and not having anyone to help.

I can remember having an important business meeting scheduled a few years ago when my nanny called in sick. My regular babysitters were all in school, and I was so stressed out, wracking my brain for what to do. I hated to cancel such an important meeting when people where flying and driving in from all over the country to attend. So I called one girlfriend whom I'd only known for a few weeks but had really connected with and offered to pay her to watch my daughter for a few hours. She laughed and said, "Don't be silly. I'd love to have Ella over."

It was the beginning of a beautiful relationship, in which we gave to and took from each other, and it always balanced out. She ended up going through a thorny and contentious divorce and needed a lot of help with her children a few months later. We became each other's backup, neither of us having our moms or family anywhere nearby. We had created our own village of love and support, and our children were better off for it.

Strategies for Developing a Support Network

Through my experiences as a military spouse, I've watched countless women go through the process of developing a support network and have done it quite a few times myself. Here are a few of my best tips for helping you develop your own network of support and love, which is sure to enrich your motherhood experience:

— Offer to trade childcare with a friend so you can take turns getting away and doing fun things by yourself. A massage or pedicure sounds much more affordable when you aren't paying for childcare, as well!

— Offer to watch a friend's child when you can tell she's in need. Essentially, you are paying it forward, hoping she might do the same for you one day. But do these things with no expectation; rather, do it out of love.

— Support networks are generally developed with a group of close friends that you really trust and bond with. Military spouses have it really easy this way; we often have numerous women to choose from who are very open because they are all in the same boat. Gyms, coffee shops, bookstores, churches, synagogues, and other religious venues are great places to meet new friends.

— I've had to move to new places, knowing nobody, seven times now in my life! It can be intimidating and tough to get used to striking up conversations with complete strangers, but such encounters have led to some of my very best friends to this day.

— Mothers of Preschoolers (MOPS) groups are all over, and through them you will meet numerous women who have something very significant in common—motherhood!

— Join a new gym that has childcare. You will be able to scope out the other moms and strike up conversations while finishing a class or working out next to each other.

— Volunteer at your child's school, and chat with the other moms. Maybe you will hit it off with one and can offer to carpool or get together for play dates.

I'd like to give you some examples of how conversations that I initiated with strangers resulted in lifelong friendships.

I saw a woman walking at the gym, and she was holding a book about Paris. I'd just gone there a few months earlier and said something like, "Are you going to Europe? Paris is one of my favorite cities!" We ended up meeting for coffee to talk about Europe before she left on her vacation. That was 12 years ago, and she's still a close friend.

A friend of a friend had been given my phone number when she moved to my town. She said she felt silly and nervous, but she got the nerve up to call me out of the blue and introduce herself. I invited her to my daughter's birthday party the next day, and she is now one of my closest friends and will be forever.

I was introduced to a neighbor's fiancée out one night at a bar. We had both just moved to Alaska and had left the jobs of our dreams in the "lower 48." We were both feeling like we'd given up so much for our men. She asked me to join her for a walk one day, and we ended up walking for two hours because we enjoyed our conversation so much. Nine years and five children later, she is still one of my dearest friends, and we talk a few times each week about everything—from raising our kids to training for marathons. She is a crucial part of my support system from afar.

A new woman had just moved to town and joined our squadron in Florida. She was about to have a baby within a few weeks. Her husband told mine that she was terribly lonely and depressed about having a baby so far from her family, which was in another country. I got together with a few other women, and we threw her a baby shower. She has been a close friend ever since.

I was on a hike with some new people when I hit it off with one woman in particular. We had both gone to the University of Minnesota. She invited me to see *The Vagina Monologues* with a group of four other women. We all became instant friends, and they are an integral part of my support network to this day.

I could go on and on . . . the point is you never know when you are going to meet your new best friend. Be open. Talk to people in places where you normally might not. Smile at people. If you chat with someone whom you bond with, ask her to meet you for coffee or to join you at a yoga class. She is probably as happy to meet you as you are to meet her.

Support networks are crucial for moms on many levels. Having a friend to talk to on a rough day is invaluable. Knowing that women will be there during tough times helps make life more livable, even on the worst days. The women in your network are the ones who will call just to see how you're doing and will bring you meals after you've had a baby. They will take your children when you're sick. It's so reassuring to know that people are looking out for you and have your back through the joys and sorrows of life.

After a devastating miscarriage, I will never forget the heavy cloak of sadness that I felt. I had to have a D&C, which is a minor procedure but pretty painful when you're already sad about losing a baby. I returned home to discover flowers, loving letters, and a voicemail from each of my best friends. I cried tears of gratitude and felt completely surrounded and soothed by their love. My three oldest and dearest hometown friends booked their tickets the moment they found out I'd lost the baby and knew I needed them. They arrived two weeks later and had arranged for us to stay at a beautiful hotel on the beach. With them, I learned I could smile and be lighthearted again. After the initial hugs and tears, we didn't mention the miscarriage again the entire trip. Instead, we went out for delicious meals and drank too many margaritas, danced until we could barely walk, and went back to our hotel room with an extra-large pizza at 3 A.M. We told stories, laughed, shopped, and relaxed at the spa. This trip literally brought me back to life.

This is what your support network will do. They are the ones who will show up at your door with your favorite dinner when you're having one of your worst days. They are the ones who will see that you're wiped out and offer to take your kids for a few hours to give you a break. These women will sustain you in the tough times, support you in your endeavors, and celebrate your joys and victories with you.

Affirmation for the Week

The happiest people in the world are those with nurturing and supportive networks of friends and family. My most important relationships require my energy and input to sustain and nurture them. I will be sure to take the time to reach out to these special people and stay connected. My life will be much more joyful for it. When I am nearing the end of my time on earth, I will remember my relationships as the most precious things in my life, not my possessions or my status in the world.

★◻★

Not Just a Mom

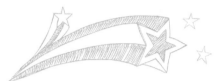

"The purpose of life is to live it, to taste experience to the utmost, to reach out eagerly and without fear for newer and richer experience."

— ELEANOR ROOSEVELT

Moms, particularly stay-at-home moms, are often reduced to thinking, *I'm just a mom.* I have heard this sentiment dozens of times from women all over the country, from all walks of life. I believe it is demeaning and greatly undervalues the essential job that mothers do in raising the next generation. Women raising children are so much more than "just moms." Don't let the labels of society and your own mind hold you back from living a life that is authentic and purposeful, whether you work outside the home or not.

My goal this week is to inspire you to look within, get clear on your life's purpose at this moment, and develop a roadmap to guide you toward your ideal life and the best version of yourself. I will coach you to spend time defining what you really want from life and then set specific, attainable tasks, goals, and deadlines to make sure you are moving toward your goal.

Life's Seasons

I want you to remember that our lives have seasons. While we may have an overarching life purpose, as we experience various stages of our lives, our primary focus changes. For example, my overarching desire has always been to make the world a better, happier place. I am most joyful when whatever I am doing is in alignment with that overall purpose.

During the eight years between finishing graduate school and having my first child, one of my purposes became my corporate job and helping my company make money. As an environmental consultant, I certainly felt like I was having a positive impact on society by improving water quality. I was usually in my office analyzing numbers and writing technical memos, so I often had to consciously make the link between what I was doing and how people were being helped. I was good at my job and enjoyed it in general, but there was always a voice inside nudging me to realize my dreams and start living them. I became a married woman during that time, and I entered the season of matrimony and maintaining a marvelous marriage—which became another one of my life's primary purposes. When we partner with the right person, he or she helps us take a step closer to living our life's purpose and helps us grow in a way that leads us to fulfill our dreams.

Then I became a mother. When I first held my oldest daughter, I realized that protecting her, loving her, and raising her to achieve her fullest potential were my new primary focuses. I had entered a new season, one that prompted me to start evaluating everything in my life on a deeper level. I hope motherhood can do the same for you. I kept working at my corporate job, but my heart and mind were more focused on my child. I enjoyed getting out of the house, dressing up, and feeling like an important adult, but after a while, I recognized it was my ego that felt it needed that job to feel good. Finally, I decided that working part-time was a much better match for what was in my heart; things instantly felt one step better in my life. My husband and I had to adjust to living on a little less, but the reduction in stress and increase in joy made it all completely worth it.

Our children are babies, toddlers, and preschoolers for such a short while. It doesn't always feel that way when we are in the middle of it, but while these children are young, they simply become one of our primary purposes for living. This does not mean a mother is all that we are. We are still who we have been and always will be. Ideally, becoming a mother prompts us to grow and to take one step closer to our highest potential. We have the power to make the world a better place, by raising happy, well-adjusted human beings. We must set the best possible example for our children by living our own very best lives.

Listening to the Voice Within

Through my first years of motherhood and even after I reduced my work to part-time, there was still a little voice within letting me know that I was not yet living in alignment with my life's purpose. This voice became louder as my corporate success grew. I was having many great accomplishments at work, making my ego believe I was irreplaceable and that my colleagues wouldn't be able to make do without me. Simultaneously, I felt more inner disharmony and longing for my daughter. When my baby lunged for her nanny, it made my heart ache, even though my logical mind was happy that she was so comfortable with her caretaker.

When I found out we were expecting another baby, I was overjoyed. Everything in my life had worked out rather smoothly and according to plan. My children would be precisely two-and-a-half years apart, just as I had envisioned. At nine weeks, we saw the baby in the ultrasound and heard its little heartbeat. The heart rate was a little slower than they would have liked, so I was asked to come back two weeks later to make sure everything was okay. I had a few moments of fear but shook it off, believing that everything would work out for the best for me—as it usually did.

Two weeks later, my husband, daughter, and I went to the ultrasound, and the technician was unable to find a heartbeat. Furthermore, she had a look of panic on her face when she said, "Excuse me. I will be right back." I knew something was terribly wrong and broke down crying. My husband comforted me the best he could, but both of us were wrecked. My wonderful doctor came in, and with a grave look, stated that unfortunately, the baby was no longer alive. Then she asked me to get dressed and meet her in her office.

After a passionate sobbing session, I pulled myself together, and we went into the doctor's office. She had printed out an ultrasound picture and showed me a picture of my uterus. Not only was there a little dead baby in my womb but a strange mass of cells, which was a quickly growing tumor. The baby would never have survived with the mass of cells taking all the nutrients. I had what's called a partial molar pregnancy. The doctor would have to perform a D&C to remove the baby and mass; then I would need to undergo weekly blood tests to make sure the tumor cells were completely removed and not regrowing. I left the office numb.

Then, the night after my D&C, I became mad. I was painfully bitter and I cried with anger in a way that I had never experienced. I was up in the middle of the night and asked, "Why me, God?" Then I felt words. I heard God, who said, "I am sad, too. I do not want to see you suffering." A sense of calm and peace came over me, and I never felt that anger again. I knew I had to use this situation to grow as a woman.

During my time of sadness and recovery, I found solace and peace in prayer and meditation. This tragic event prompted me to wake up early and take time to meditate every morning. This practice has changed my life for the better, and now I hear my inner voice much more clearly. Once you hear your inner voice clearly, it becomes hard to ignore.

Six months of blood testing revealed that the tumor was not going to come back, and we were given the go-ahead to try for another baby. I quickly became pregnant. My second pregnancy, until shortly after the birth of my second daughter, was a time of great growth for me. Some of the growth was painful, such as when I finally faced that things weren't perfect in my marriage— and we had to make some great strides toward reconnecting and strengthening our relationship. During that experience, my inner voice told me that the way I was living my life was not in alignment with God's purpose for me. This became more and more apparent, and I was just waiting for the right time to make the major changes I needed to.

Listen to the voice while it is still a whisper. Take the time to pay attention. When you have a thought that keeps coming into your mind, over and over, or a feeling of exceeding joy or utter dissatisfaction, listen. Your inner voice is clearly trying to tell you something important!

What Does Success Mean to You?

An important idea to ponder is what success means to you. If you feel most successful at your job, where you feel appreciated, fulfilled, and "on purpose," then working might be a part of the happiness equation for you as a mother. There is nothing wrong with working while raising children, especially if your work brings you great satisfaction and joy. I am now working a few hours a week as an environmental consultant and as an author, and it rarely adds too much stress to my life.

Does success to you mean security and making a lot of money? If so, do the sacrifices required to make a lot of money sit well within your heart? If the answer is yes to both questions, then that's what you need to do. To some people, financial security is an overarching need required for their greatest happiness. To others, having a primary role in raising their babies is the most important measure of success, and money is secondary. These people will make the sacrifices necessary to live on less in order to achieve their ideal of success.

I feel the most successful when I am living in balance, pursuing my own creative endeavors, but spending what feels like the right amount of time with my husband and children. I feel successful when my house is fairly neat and my refrigerator is stocked so that I can make healthy, delicious meals. I can tell you this certainly has not always been my definition of success, but these days it's what does it for me.

So what does success mean to you? Now that you are a mother, your definition may have changed. Some days, getting up, dressed, and to the gym with a young baby may be considered a rousing success! Other days, seeing that your baby has put on weight may give you the most gratitude you have had in a while. At one time, getting an outstanding raise at work indicated success to me; but after my kids were born, that measure of success lost a lot of its appeal. I knew I couldn't take time away from my family to achieve corporate success in the same way I once did.

Don't Hide

Many moms that I talk to and work with say they have hidden behind their role as a mom, using it as an excuse for losing touch with their dreams. It's easy to see how the consuming role of motherhood can take us further and further from our dream life, causing us to lose touch with our inner voice. The task of getting back in connection with ourselves is not easy, and any mom knows that the path of least resistance is to lose sight of what is deep within her, longing to be expressed.

Stop hiding. Your journey as a mom should not stop your quest for personal growth and individual success.

Labels

Along the journey of self-discovery, we realize that we have put many labels on ourselves. These labels indicate how we identify ourselves. Some of the labels bring us great pride; others, not so much. I know many women whose identities were so wrapped up in their titles or positions (including myself) that the transition to mother was tough. It was in their hearts to cut back on their professional lives and stay home with their children for a while. But the roughest part was being asked what they did, and replying, "I'm a stay-at-home mom."

Many women say this as though it is a diminished status or position. One friend told me she always utters it with a sense of shame because at one point, she was so proud of her role as a TV personality. It's easy to become identified with our position and equate our personal importance with our professional title. In a society that often prizes possessions and power, it is easy to see why women don't always feel proud to say, "I am a mother, and I stay home with my kids." Most stay-at-home moms have countless other options, but they choose to make their children their priority. There is no shame in that.

If you identify with your position or role, your work becomes so much a part of who you are that it can be extraordinarily difficult to separate yourself from it. For some women, their life's work is their current job, and having children is simply a joyful addition. This is a choice, and this lifestyle can be led with just as much love and joy as any other. Children of mothers who work full-time or part-time can be just as happy, well-adjusted, and fabulous as those of stay-at-home moms. As long as a mother is living in alignment with her life's primary purpose, she is setting the best possible example for her children—no matter what label the world gives her.

What's Holding You Back?

So, what is stopping you from achieving your goals? You are in control of your life, no matter what you think. You have the power to make real whatever it is you desire. The only thing holding you back is your own thinking. Maybe you can't achieve the end goal you have in mind while caring for a new baby, but you can continue to dream and to become clearer on what you really desire. You can set smaller goals and take baby steps to research your dream. Becoming a mother should not prevent you from taking some form of action to keep moving forward.

Your Thinking

Is your thinking holding you back? We all have a number of excuses for why we aren't living or moving toward our ideal life. They are simply excuses, and every human uses them at one point or another. I had a list of excuses that I used when it came to actually quitting my corporate job. In fact, I am still technically an employee of that company, on an hourly flex status. I really haven't released it completely. It's hard to let go of a comfortable situation, even when your rational mind knows it's not helping you move toward your highest potential.

Your Financial Situation

Is your financial situation holding you back? This excuse is one that can be very real, and very stressful. In order to fund basic living expenses, many of us feel as though we have to work at a job that is secure and pays well. This is understandable, but you still have to follow your dreams to live life to its fullest. Perform beautifully at whatever job you have at the moment, knowing that it doesn't have to be forever. Do it with class, exceed expectations, and learn whatever you can. This part of your life may be a crucial personal experience, giving you something you need for greatness later. You can still dream. You can still set goals for yourself and make progress toward a more comfortable financial situation.

Your Fear

Is your fear holding you back? Fear, in some form or another, is a big block for many of us. We all have fears that prevent us from pursuing what we really want in life. The idea is to recognize our fears, neutralize them, and move forward. In every situation where I doubt my own abilities, I think, *What is the very worst that could happen? Would my family still be there, safe and sound?* If the answer is yes, I imagine myself handling the worst outcome with grace. This exercise counteracts my fears and helps me take huge leaps of faith. I do the thing I fear, knowing it will help me make great strides forward.

Fear is natural and can help protect us in some situations. The problem is that our brains often start generating fear of things simply because they are daring, different, or pushing us out of our comfort zone. Evaluate your fear. Determine if it is warranted or simply a part of you that needs to grow and be pushed outside its place of ease.

Your Life Circumstances

When I want to succumb to my own excuses, I think of Tererai Trent. Tererai was a guest on an episode of *The Oprah Winfrey Show* that I just happened to watch recorded one evening. Tererai is from Zimbabwe, where she grew up in abject poverty in a culture that did not value girls enough to allow them to have an education. She learned to read and write by doing her brother's schoolwork, before being married off at the age of 11. This woman was inspired by an American employee of Heifer International to believe that she could dare to dream.

And dream she did. Tererai has achieved every lofty goal she has set for herself. She made it to the United States, undergoing beatings every day by her husband until he was deported for abuse. She went on to raise five children as a single mother while earning her bachelor's degree, her master's degree, and finally, her Ph.D. If this woman can overcome unimaginable adversity to achieve such greatness, just imagine what people with lesser hardships can accomplish. What sets Tererai apart? She became clear on her dreams, wrote them down, and believed fully that it was possible to achieve them. And so she did.

Our motivation and belief in ourselves will go up and down throughout our lives. But hopefully, as we get older, wiser, and more confident, we will realize that we truly can make things happen. Sure, there will be setbacks, but these are simply learning and strengthening experiences in the process. Have you ever noticed that those who achieve the most amazing things have also often undergone some of the most difficult life circumstances? Hard times only make us stronger and more suited for our ultimate life's purpose. Sometimes these difficulties are just the thing to prepare us for the next thing, which is going to be bigger and better than the last.

Dreaming and Setting Goals

I found motherhood to be the perfect opportunity to evaluate my existence on a deeper level and take the time to dream about what I truly wanted to do with my life. Was my career bringing me real joy and satisfaction? What did I envision doing to make a difference in the world, and how could I balance this goal with caring for my family? I realized that I had no idea. I needed to become clear on what I really wanted out of life.

Becoming Clear

One of the first things we must do to set and achieve goals is to become clear as to what our dreams are. This is often one of the toughest parts of the process because many of us have stopped allowing ourselves to think big. We may have accepted our lot in life and decided it's easier just to continue moving forward, day by day, without keeping the larger picture in mind. When was the last time you actually sat down and thought about what you really wanted out of your human experience? Knowing you only get one shot at it, what do you really want to do with your life?

I want you to carve out a few minutes this week to brainstorm about your dreams. You can do this while you are exercising or quietly feeding your baby. It's your life, and this exercise is important. Here are a few questions I want you to ask yourself to help you start developing a clearer picture as to what you are all about. Get out a pen and paper if it helps you to write things down (it helps me!):

- What things have you done in your life that have made you feel the most alive and joyful?

- What activities do you "lose yourself" in so that time flies by and you get completely engrossed?

- If money was absolutely not an issue, what would you do differently in your life?

- What is your ideal life?

- How does your ideal life differ from your current reality?

- What could you achieve in your life that would make you think, *Wow, I've really made it*?

- Can you think of any small steps you could take, starting today, toward your dream life?

If You Believe It, You Can Achieve It

I believe this with all my heart. You might be in a place in your life where you just want to be home, focusing on your baby and living a peaceful and simple life. If this is what brings you joy and feels right to you, then it's exactly what you should do. If part of you is longing to do something a little more (perhaps something you discovered during the exercise in the previous section), then it's time to start setting some goals for yourself. Don't be intimidated by setting goals. Here are a few things to keep in mind:

- Goals should be broken down into doable pieces.

- Goals should be realistic.

- Goals should be very clear and precise.

- Goals should be smaller steps leading you to a greater goal.

- Goals should have a schedule and deadline associated with them that are achievable, considering your life situation.

Think of your goals as a way you can get excited about your future and feel like you are taking action. A goal can be as simple as, "I am going to spend one hour this week researching graduate schools." And the next week, "I am going to select three schools to investigate further and determine admissions requirements." And then maybe a month or two later, "I am going to submit applications to my top three universities." The point is, if there is something inside you that you'd like to accomplish or a dream you'd like to realize, feel empowered now to take tiny steps toward achieving it.

I believe in you, but you have to believe in yourself. The sheer magnitude of time and energy required to care for a newborn can zap your confidence that you can still achieve greatness. You can. In fact, as a mother, you can accomplish anything that you could have before—and more.

Nourishment: Carbohydrates

Carbohydrates are much more fascinating and complicated than previously thought, and nutrition researchers are continuing to learn new things. Carbohydrates are one of the three main classes of foods, which also include fats and proteins. Carbohydrates are used for energy in the body and are organic compounds that are comprised of sugars, starches, and fiber. A lot of emphasis is put on reducing carbohydrates when dieting because if a carbohydrate isn't burned off or used soon after it is consumed, a small portion is stored in the muscles and your liver as glycogen (for energy), and the rest will be stored in your body as fat.

Here is more information about the various types of carbohydrates.

Simple Sugars

Sugar is ubiquitous in the American diet. Therefore, it is important to understand the nutritional aspects of sugar to protect your health and achieve your ideal weight. The primary forms of sugar include monosaccharides, disaccharides, and oligosaccharides.

Monosaccharides and Disaccharides (Sugars or Simple Carbohydrates). Monosaccharides are the simplest sugars and are the building blocks of larger carbohydrates. Monosaccharides are the only carbohydrates that can be directly absorbed into the bloodstream through the intestines. Disaccharides result from the combination of two monosaccharide molecules. A common example is table sugar, also known as sucrose, which is the combination of one molecule of fructose and one molecule of sucrose.

Oligosaccharides. Oligosaccharides function more akin to fiber, and typically contain two to ten monosaccharide molecules. They are found naturally in wheat, leeks, onions, asparagus, chicory root, legumes, soybeans, and Jerusalem artichokes. They can be synthesized in the body from lactose (milk sugar). Oligosaccharides have been drawing the interest of the nutrition community due to their newly discovered purpose as a prebiotic. The human body has a difficult time breaking down many oligosaccharides (and other prebiotics), which means a majority of them make their way into the colon. There, they promote the growth of beneficial bacteria. (Resistant starches and fermentable fiber are also prebiotics.)

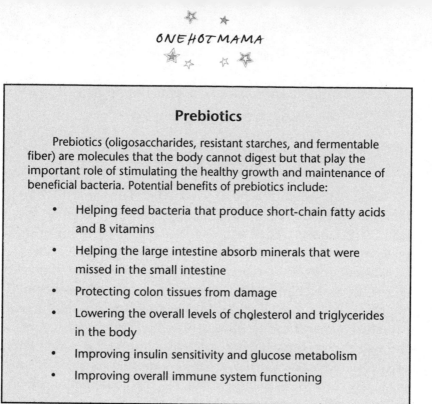

Prebiotics

Prebiotics (oligosaccharides, resistant starches, and fermentable fiber) are molecules that the body cannot digest but that play the important role of stimulating the healthy growth and maintenance of beneficial bacteria. Potential benefits of prebiotics include:

- Helping feed bacteria that produce short-chain fatty acids and B vitamins
- Helping the large intestine absorb minerals that were missed in the small intestine
- Protecting colon tissues from damage
- Lowering the overall levels of cholesterol and triglycerides in the body
- Improving insulin sensitivity and glucose metabolism
- Improving overall immune system functioning

The Downside of a Diet High in Sugar

Sugar has become omnipresent in the American diet. Here are a few statistics that highlight the extent of the sugar-consumption problem in our culture:[1]

- In 1800, the average person consumed about 18 pounds of sugar per year.
- In 1890, the obesity rate based on one study was 3.4 percent.
- In 1900, the average person consumed 90 pounds of sugar per year.
- In 2009, more than half of the American population consumed 180 pounds of sugar each year.
- In 2010, 33.8 percent of Americans were obese.[2]

More specifically, we consume far too much fructose, which is a form of sugar that wreaks significantly more havoc on our bodies than glucose (think high-fructose corn syrup, which is found in so many food products!). Fructose elevates uric acid in your body, which has many dangerous side effects, such as raising your blood pressure and damaging your kidneys. It can cause chronic, low-level inflammation in your body. Fructose messes with your body's metabolism because it does not suppress the hormone ghrelin (which makes you feel hungry), and it does not stimulate the release of leptin (which makes you feel satisfied) in the proper proportions, which basically makes you want to eat more.

Here are some compelling reasons why we should really cut back on sugar:[3]

- Sugar can cause premature aging and a decrease in tissue elasticity (i.e., more sagging and wrinkling).

- Sugar feeds cancer cells.

- Excess sugar consumption is linked to autoimmune diseases, such as arthritis, asthma, and multiple sclerosis.

- Sugar can cause tooth decay and gum disease.

- Excess sugar can exacerbate hemorrhoids and varicose veins.

- High sugar intake can decrease your insulin sensitivity and eventually lead to diabetes.

- Sugar can damage your DNA, liver, kidneys, pancreas, and adrenal glands.

- Sugar can exacerbate depression.

- Sugar can cause fluid retention (which none of us wants!).

Starches

Starches, also known as polysaccharides and complex carbohydrates, are longer and more complex chains of monosaccharides. Starches include grains (wheat, rice, barley, and oats), potatoes, corn, and beans. It has been commonly believed that complex carbohydrates do not raise blood sugar as quickly as simpler sugars. However, we now know that some starches break down very quickly and cause a bigger spike in blood sugar (rapidly digested starch [RDS]), while others are digested more slowly and do not impact blood sugar as dramatically (slowly digested starch [SDS]). It is important to note that the larger the percentage of rapidly digested starch in a food, the higher its glycemic index (GI). The third type of starch, resistant starch, is not digested in the small intestine; it acts as a prebiotic, similar to oligosaccharides and fermentable fiber.

Glycemic Index (GI)

This number ranks carbohydrates according to the impact that a food has on our blood sugar levels. Lower-GI carbohydrates produce a smaller spike in our blood's glucose and insulin levels. Low-GI diets have benefits such as keeping you full longer, reducing heart disease, and enhancing physical endurance.

Fiber

Fiber, like other carbohydrates, is made up of monosaccharide molecules. It is the part of a plant that is not digestible by humans. Therefore, fiber passes through the digestive tract without being broken down and absorbed into the bloodstream. There are essentially three types of fiber:

Soluble Fiber. This form of fiber absorbs and retains water like a sponge, creating a gel-like substance that slows digestion and in the process, stabilizes blood sugar and allows your body to better absorb nutrients from your food. Soluble fiber reduces your cholesterol. It also tends to make you feel full, so you won't want to eat as much when consuming foods with soluble fiber, which include beans, oatmeal, citrus, carrots, apples, berries, nuts, seeds, and flax.

Insoluble Fiber. Insoluble fiber is the "roughage" that we usually associate with the word *fiber*. It keeps things moving and prevents constipation. Whole wheat, wheat bran, and vegetables are good sources of insoluble fiber.

Fermentable Fiber. Fermentable fiber is also indigestible, but it acts as a very useful prebiotic to keep your digestive system healthier and to potentially boost your immune system. Fermentable fiber includes pectin, which is found in berries and apples. Fermentable fiber is also found in oats, bananas, prebiotic yogurt, leafy green vegetables (such as spinach, collard greens, and kale), and whole grains.

The Benefits of Fiber

There are many benefits of a high-fiber diet, which will help women in the process of losing their baby weight. These benefits include the following:

- Fiber helps keep your digestive system healthy and your bowels normal.

- Fiber lowers the cholesterol levels in your blood.

- Fiber reduces your blood pressure and the overall inflammation in your body.

- Fiber stabilizes and controls blood sugar levels by slowing the absorption of sugar into your bloodstream.

- Fiber helps with weight loss because a high-fiber diet makes you feel full faster and keeps you satisfied longer.

The Carbohydrate Bottom Line

In this section, we learned about the important types of carbohydrates, including simple sugars, starches, and fiber. The three most important take-home messages are:

1. Reduce your sugar consumption.

2. Maintain healthy starches in your diet, including beans; lentils; and whole grains, such as brown rice, barley, and quinoa (which are slowly digested or resistant starch).

3. Minimize processed foods, such as sugary cereals and baked goods made with white flour.

Fitness: Exercising for Happiness

As a mom, I can attest that working out is one of the most important things for maintaining my mental clarity and inner peace. Honestly, I can start a run in the absolute worst mood, stressed out and cranky, and by the time I am done, I have sweated it out to the point that I am calm and happy. One long walk with a friend and I have not only connected with someone I care about, but I have usually talked about some things that have been stressing me out, have gotten my heart rate up, and am feeling free and fabulous. One study performed at the University of Texas showed that depressed participants reported feeling much happier and more vibrant after a 30-minute walk.[4]

Many moms struggle with feelings of depression from time to time. They are exhausted, overwhelmed, lonely, and just plain down. Depressed people generally have lower levels of neurotransmitters, such as serotonin and norepinephrine, in their brains. These neurotransmitters make you feel balanced and happy and stabilize your mood by soothing anxiety. Exercise stimulates the sympathetic nervous system, which causes these "happiness and well-being" neurotransmitters to flow into your body.[5]

After her husband was deployed to Afghanistan, my dear friend Jess became a runner. Her runs were one of the few times during the day when she could be alone with her thoughts, since she was home full-time, alone, with two preschool-aged children. She wrote to me about how important her runs became during this time:

> I could plan out my week, pray, listen to music, or daydream about what he was doing at that same moment. I could let my mind focus on the run and nothing else. Conversely, I could let my thoughts wander and propel me through a challenging trail. I felt centered, ready for my next challenge, physically strengthened, and emotionally grounded. I also felt empowered to take on the challenges of being a "single" mom. Let's face it: If you can run 12 miles in the snow before your kids are even awake, you can do anything!

It is a proven fact that exercising can help keep your mind and body balanced and healthy, but it is also an escape. Like Jess, I use my exercise time to enjoy unfettered thinking or simple peace and quiet. Sometimes, my brain just has to run through the laundry list of things that have been bothering me. When my life is hectic and my brain just can't keep up with everything, my exercise time is when these things just organize and file themselves.

In Week 7's workout schedule, below, we continue to make very small additions of time each day. Please increase the challenge of your workouts as you feel ready and in shape enough to do so. Sometimes we see the scale stop moving downward because we aren't pushing ourselves in our workouts. This week, add a little intensity to a workout or two, or pick up the pace!

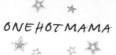
Week 7 Workout Schedule

Monday	Tuesday	Wednesday	Thursday	Friday	Saturday	Sunday
45-minute walk or 30-minute jog	30 minutes strength	1-hour walk, 30-minute jog, or cardio class at gym	30 minutes strength	45-minute walk, 30-minute jog, or cardio class at gym	Yoga or Pilates class	Rest

The "No Mom-Butt Here" Workout

Before this workout, do a five-minute warm-up to make sure your muscles are loosened up. Jog around the house, or do some jumping jacks. Shake your booty, and make it fun!

1. *Bridge Lift.* Start by lying flat on your back on a mat, with your knees bent and your arms at your sides. Raise your pelvis toward the ceiling, flexing your buttocks as hard as you can, to a point where your body will be at about a 45-degree angle relative to the floor. Hold for a few counts, return to the ground, and repeat 20 to 25 times.

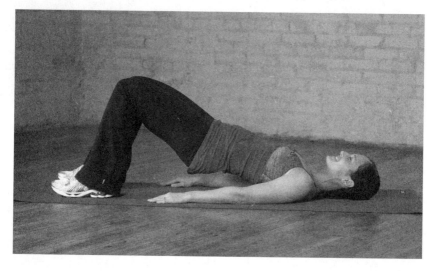

2. *Squat Dips.* Lift your left leg and place it on top of a chair about three feet behind you. Lower into a single-leg squat, making sure your knee does not extend past your toes. Straighten your right leg to stand. Do 15 repetitions, and then switch legs and repeat.

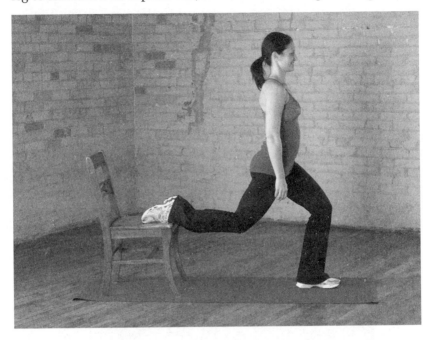

3. *Curtsy Lunge.* Start with your feet approximately hip-width apart and then lunge your right leg behind your body and to the left, just like a curtsy. As you cross your leg behind, bend both knees until your left quadriceps is almost parallel to the floor. Be sure to keep your core engaged. Return to the starting position by using your muscles to straighten your legs back to standing. Feel free to add a weight or hold your baby for a greater challenge. Perform 10 to 15 repetitions on your right leg, and then switch legs.

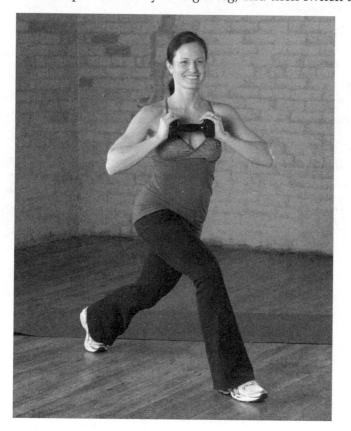

4. *Butt Kickers (Donkey Kicks).* Start down on all fours. Lift your right leg to hip height with foot flexed, knee bent to 90 degrees. Lift your leg toward the ceiling, foot flat. Repeat 25 times, and then switch sides and repeat.

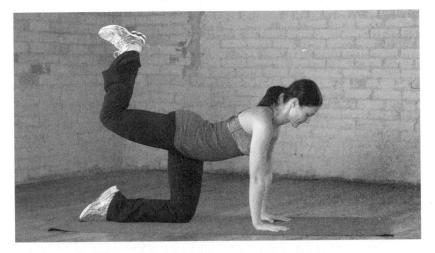

5. *Fire Hydrant Lifts.* Start down on all fours. Engage your core, and slowly lift your right leg out to the side until it's parallel to the floor, keeping it bent at a 90-degree angle. Repeat 15 to 25 times on one side and then switch legs.

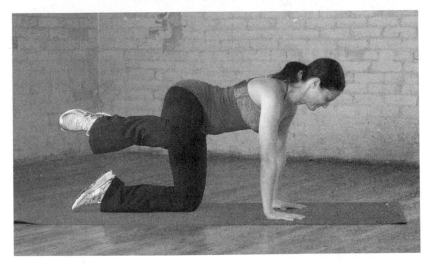

Sanity Saver: Guilty Pleasures

An easy way for moms to add a little fun and joy to their lives is by partaking in a guilty pleasure. What is a guilty pleasure? It's an enjoyable activity that you recognize as a treat. It's something a little low-brow or that probably shouldn't be done for hours a day. A guilty pleasure is something that makes you feel a little spoiled. It's usually something you don't "need" in life, but it makes you smile and gives you a little respite from the often over-whelming and mundane activities of caring for a baby, home, and other responsibilities.

Moms give, give, and give some more, so taking a little time to be completely indulgent and selfish is part of rebalancing, in my opinion. At the end of a particularly trying day, I relish putting my feet up for a few minutes and watching some mindless TV with a glass of wine. Catching up on fashion and gossip magazines while getting a pedicure is another great way to do something just for yourself, to regain your sense of humor and reclaim your joy. There are so many opportunities each day for you to steal a few moments for yourself; and really, there's no reason at all to feel guilty. Here are a few no-guilt, guilty pleasure suggestions:

- Lounging in the tub with a steamy novel
- The *Twilight* books and movies
- Shopping
- Celebrity gossip shows and websites
- Pinterest, fashion blogs, YouTube, Facebook, Twitter, and other addictive social media sites
- A square of dark chocolate dipped in peanut butter
- A large skinny mocha sipped slowly
- Watching a little mindless TV, such as *The Real Housewives, American Idol, Grey's Anatomy,* or *Tosh.0*

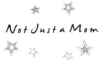

- Getting a pedicure with a girlfriend, and sipping on a latte or a glass of wine while doing so

- Making a delicious meal just for yourself

- Getting a babysitter so you can sit alone at a coffee shop and write, read, or simply be

While these are technically "guilty pleasures," for moms I actually consider them crucial re-centering activities. Guilty pleasures do not have to cost money, but getting an indulgent massage can make you feel right with the world again after a rough week at home with a baby. Just make sure to do something completely pampering that brings you a bit of joy, not caring what anyone in the world thinks of it. Nobody needs to know anyway!

Affirmation for the Week

Motherhood is the most life-changing and important role I will ever take on. However, I am still myself, and I have many talents to share with the world. I am still fun, interesting, and sexy. I have a deeper purpose, which will be fulfilled while raising children. When I use my unique gifts and talents to make the world a better place, I am living in alignment with my purpose, and I am living my very best life possible. When I live with intention, I not only feel more fulfilled, but I am also setting the best example for my children.

★❑★

The Power of Motherhood

"Of all the rights of women, the greatest is to be a mother."

— LIN YUTANG

What an enormous gift and duty it is to love and raise children. It is a role that cannot be taken lightly, for the influence we have on our children every day cannot be understated. The way we behave and handle every situation is setting a model for our children. Even as babies, they are watching our every move and are learning how to be in the world. Infants as young as two and three weeks old already have the ability to mimic simple facial movements, while babies in their second year of life will try to copy everything you do.[1]

Motherhood can make you a better person overall, and I have seen countless women softened and enlightened by the experience. Why? I believe we start to see humanity in a new light, viewing life as more beautiful and profound than before. We experience carrying a child within us who becomes completely unique and special. We watch that newborn slowly morph into an independent little person who is fresh and innocent, wanting to learn everything about the world through us. Parenting is powerful, and we have the ability to guide another human being through the tender and vulnerable first years of life.

Can Motherhood Make You a Better or More Joyful Person?

It depends. The stresses and demands of motherhood can push you either way; it seems to bring out the best and worst in people. I have seen myself remain calm and loving in the most stressful, horrible parenting conditions; I have also broken down and yelled at one of my daughters during a stressful situation when I wasn't at my best. Motherhood can certainly be a great opportunity for personal growth in areas such as patience, compassion, and unconditional love.

Why don't you try to use the experience of motherhood to elevate yourself in all areas of your life? As I have said, our children mimic our behavior in every way, including how we eat, live, talk, treat others, treat ourselves, and respond to stressors. We should use the experience of raising children to raise our personal standards, setting the best possible example. Instead of becoming a "boring" parent, use the experience to become most fully and beautifully yourself.

Motherhood Can Make You More Compassionate and Empathetic

Babies are helpless sponges of love. All they want is to be cared for and nourished with attention. Most women naturally become more compassionate and empathetic after becoming mothers. Of course, there are many times when we need to soothe, hold, and simply love our children. We are the primary builders of their self-esteem, and we have the ability to bring them up to realize their full potential.

I believe that in most cases, this sense of compassion and empathy extends beyond our relationship with our children. We can use it to help make the world a better place. Mothers are kind and generous with other moms and other children, and this benevolence can extend to all of humanity when we are at our best.

Motherhood Can Make You Happier Overall

Children are helpless and require continual attention, which can leave us feeling drained. The weight of paying for and raising human beings can be stressful, too. But when motherhood is good, it is absolutely blissful. As a mother, the highs are much higher. This morning I was in my overstuffed chair with a daughter cuddled up to me in each arm, and my heart swelled to fill my chest. The open, innocent, and complete love that children are capable of giving is one of the most beautiful things to experience. When you see your child's bright and shiny smile after a bath or watch your children express their silly side, you will feel a raw form of joy.

Children are fun, too. Sometimes we adults tend to be a little serious and forget how to just let go and laugh. I love taking the time to sit and play with my children. I don't do it as much as I'd like, but when I do, we all end up having so much fun. I also love observing the things that make my children laugh. My younger daughter went through a peekaboo stage for quite some time, and I could make her laugh anytime, anywhere, with any rendition of the game. Her jack-o'-lantern smile could make anyone laugh. My oldest child is more serious, but when she giggles, it is the sweetest, most precious—and contagious—sound. Babies start to smile very early, and there's not much that gives new parents more pleasure than seeing their baby's adorable, gummy grin.

Children and babies are 100 percent in the present moment. They live life fully engaged, which we adults often neglect to do. Being completely present with others gives them the gift of your true self. Babies simply enjoy living moment to moment, not worrying about what the next hour will bring. Motherhood can turn women into worrywarts, which is a known waste of energy and effort. Focusing your attention on the things you can change and actions you can take is a better way to channel your power. Use your baby to help you learn to revel in life at the moment, for it is really all we are guaranteed.

Motherhood Can Help You Bond with Other Moms

I have traveled with my children since they were weeks old, which is a reality of life when you are a military spouse. One thing that has always stood out to me is how most people will sit and watch you struggle to get your suitcase into the overhead bin, while carrying a few-months-old baby in your other arm, often with small children grabbing at your legs. Once in a while, a real gentleman will step up and help with the bags; but more often than not, it's another mother who comes to my rescue. I have had mothers with grown children offer to hold my baby while I took my older children to the lavatory, or who have gone out of their way to help entertain my restless toddlers.

Mothers understand the difficulties and complications that babies and kids can cause; therefore, we tend to be warm and more compassionate toward other mothers. We are comfortable with children and are not afraid to step in when we can see a fellow mom struggling. When you are grappling with a fussy baby while out and about, it will be the other mothers who offer you empathetic, understanding looks—while the rest of the population gives you an annoyed "shut that baby up" kind of glare.

Motherhood is an exclusive, protective club. So when you are dealing with a terrible diaper and run out of wipes, look no further than your nearest mom to be rescued—whether you know her or not. When you are home with a fussy baby and are about to lose your mind, call your best mom-friend for support. Not only will she tell you how she's been there, but she might even offer some suggestions that you hadn't thought of yet. When you're having trouble with nursing, bleeding nipples, or a barfing baby, only one who has been there will be interested and sympathetic.

Motherhood may bond you even closer to your girlfriends, sisters, and mother. I discovered a greater connection with these women in my life, whom I already loved so much, after I became a mother. Once you become a mother, you understand the other women in your life on a deeper level. Those traits of your mom's that were once overbearing become completely understandable.

Your sister-in-law, who is a naptime Nazi with her kids, used to strike you rigid but now seems wise and orderly.

Our children are a great new tool for meeting other women. When we are younger, we have numerous avenues to make friends. As we become adults, however, it can be more difficult to meet people. Even a baby can enjoy a swing at the park, where you might have the opportunity to strike up a conversation with another interesting or hip-looking mom. Participating in other activities, such as stroller fitness, baby gym, and music classes, can be an excellent way to meet new women.

We love our children so profoundly that we cannot imagine the horror of something bad happening to them. Seeing mothers in developing countries helplessly holding their starving and sick children is now nearly unbearable. Not being able to feed or care for our children due to circumstances beyond our control also seems unimaginable. My heart has grown bigger, and I believe there is a deeper level of compassion and love that most moms experience.

Motherhood Can Make You More Health Conscious

I have always been a pretty health-conscious person but would still have treats around the house for when my husband and I had cravings. When I became a parent, I felt the need to be very aware of what my baby was eating. When I read the labels of some "baby foods," especially snacks, I found them to be very processed and full of sugar. It was disappointing, but I realized that I had to take responsibility for what I fed my child. Motherhood can make us want to learn more about organic foods and the healthiest choices to protect our innocent and pure babies. This is tougher as they grow to preschool age, but I certainly look at everything I buy with more scrutiny.

Nourishment: Eating for Energy

Simply put, we eat food to give us the energy to live. Food sustains us and keeps us alive. Food is not a medication, a distraction, or a salve. While it can comfort us and we should enjoy it, we need to remember that the food we put in our mouths is what the body uses to build and recover itself. The life force of the food you eat transfers directly to your body. There are even people who believe we need to be aware of the way in which we kill the animals we eat, because the energy of the death experience transfers to us as we eat them. Consuming foods filled with vitamins, essential fatty acids, iron, and other minerals will make us feel vibrant and alive. Eating foods full of trans fats and preservatives will, in fact, slowly kill us.

There is a huge range in the benefits received from various foods. I just want to remind you to ask yourself the following before you put any food in your mouth: "Will this make me feel good? Will this make me feel healthy?" You might say that eating a huge bowl of ice cream will make you feel good, and if it's something you do only on occasion, then I agree. However, if a bowl of ice cream becomes a nightly necessity, then it's no longer a treat and you really have to think about whether it's making you feel good in the long run. If you are eating a Big Mac and fries, you know it might make you feel good momentarily; but shortly after, you might feel sluggish and have some gastrointestinal issues. I can say with certainty that fast food will not make you healthy. I think there can be a place for every type of food in our lives if we choose, but we need to eat in a way that is good for us and makes us feel healthy a majority of the time.

Here are a few useful tips to help you eat for optimal energy levels:

— Eat smaller meals more frequently to stabilize your blood sugar and keep yourself from becoming too hungry—and then overeating. Try eating three smaller meals and two snacks during the day. Awesome snacks for energy include a handful of walnuts or almonds, an apple, a hard-boiled egg, a whole wheat English muffin with peanut butter, carrots, edamame, and Greek yogurt.

— Be sure to get enough iron in your diet. Many women become anemic after giving birth; therefore it's crucial to have a high-iron diet to prevent the horribly energy-drained, weighted-down feeling of anemia. Anemia occurs when you have a lower than normal number of red blood cells in your body; you are unable to get enough oxygen to your organs and tissues, making you feel worn out. You are at a higher risk of anemia if you are not nursing, because you are likely to start your period much sooner. Foods that are high in iron include red meat, egg yolks, dark leafy greens (such as spinach), artichokes, iron-enriched cereals and grains, oysters, clams, scallops, beans, lentils, soybeans, and dried fruits (such as raisins). Consider taking supplements, as well, if you are in any way susceptible to anemia.

— Drink a lot of water, especially if you are nursing. Dehydration is one of the leading causes of fatigue and is one of the easiest conditions to fix. Keep a large water bottle nearby at all times, and remember to have a big glass of water after every feeding if you're nursing.

— Include protein and complex carbohydrates with every meal.

— Be sure you are getting enough healthy fats, especially omega-3 fatty acids, which can be harder to get in the typical American diet.

Fitness: Start Training for Something

The way I have lost the last bit of baby weight after each baby was to sign up for a running race or a triathlon (or both). In fact, I signed up for a triathlon with my husband when my second child was two months old. It was a sprint triathlon, and I did it mainly to impress my husband and to bond with him. I didn't really think it through, though, as I had not swum a lap in over three years. The afternoon before, I started realizing what I had done. I tried on my athletic swimsuit, which was a two-piece. The sight of myself about made me gag, so I got in the car and drove to the local swimsuit boutique, where they helped me find a suit that would flatter. I ended up with one that my grandmother would have loved, designed to "minimize" the midsection.

I woke up early that morning and nursed the baby right before heading out the door. Thankfully, one of my best friends was visiting, and she stayed with my daughters. As I stood on the beach, ready to jump into the Gulf of Mexico, I was filled with a mix of body consciousness, pure elation, and pride that I was doing such a crazy thing. Nobody stared at me with disgust, like I half expected them to. The swim nearly killed me, but the bike ride was fun, and by the run, I was getting into the groove. I was exhilarated but exhausted when I crossed the finish line, and I had to rush home to ease my bursting breasts.

I am more of a runner, so signing up for a race is a feasible and fun thing for me to do. I recommend waiting to train hard with running until your baby turns six months, if you are nursing, to protect your milk production. At about six to eight months, I like to start training for a 10K or a half marathon. The more ambitious can train for a marathon, while new runners can plan on doing a 5K.

If you decide running is something you'd like to do more of, you can substitute runs for all of the cardio workouts listed in the workout schedule below. But be sure to continue to get in your strength and yoga/Pilates workouts when you can, to keep your body limber, balanced, and injury free!

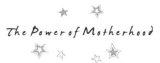
Week 8 Workout Schedule

Monday	Tuesday	Wednesday	Thursday	Friday	Saturday	Sunday
45-minute walk or 30-minute jog	30 minutes strength	1-hour walk, 30-minute jog, or cardio class at gym	30 minutes strength	45-minute walk, 30-minute jog, or cardio class at gym	Yoga or Pilates class	Rest

The "Get Rid of Your Mommy Tummy" Ab Workout

Circuit workouts are incredibly effective at helping your body get in shape more quickly, because you are continually switching exercises and keeping your heart rate up.

1. *Mountain Climbers.* To warm up, do mountain climbers by starting in a push-up position with your hands on the floor, about shoulder-width apart. Your weight will be on your hands while you bend your right knee forward to your chest and then back out straight. Quickly switch and bring in your left knee forward to your chest. It is like doing high knees but down on the floor, somewhat like the movement of hiking up a mountain! Alternate knees forward for 25 to 30 repetitions.

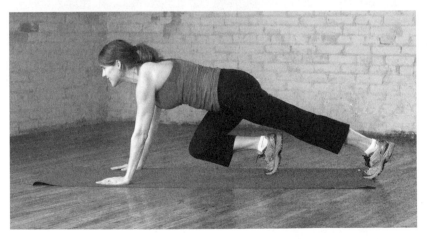

2. *Crunches.* Lie on the floor with your knees bent and your hands across your chest or behind your neck. Pull your belly button toward your spine, and bring your lower back to the floor. Contracting your abdominals, lift your shoulders a few inches off the floor, and hold for a few seconds. Slowly lower back down, but don't relax your muscles. Repeat 15 to 25 times.

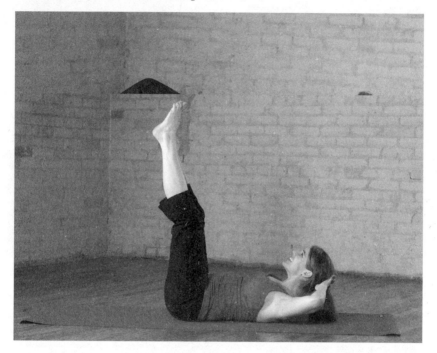

4. *Reverse Vertical Leg Crunches.* Lie on your back with your legs extended upward, knees slightly bent, with feet together or crossed. Contract your abs to lift the hips off the floor, reaching your legs up toward the ceiling. Be sure that you are using your muscles and are not using your legs for momentum. Lower and repeat 15 to 25 times.

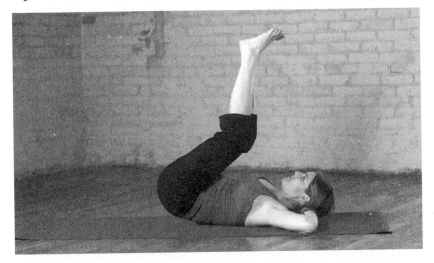

5. *Oblique Twists with a Weight (or a Baby).* Sit on the floor with your knees bent and feet flat on the floor, and then lower your upper body, keeping your back straight, until you are at a 45-degree angle. Hold the weight (or the baby) directly out in front of you. Using your abdominal muscles, twist slowly to your right, and lower the weight close to the floor. Smoothly contract your abs and twist your torso to touch the weight to the other side. Repeat 15 times.

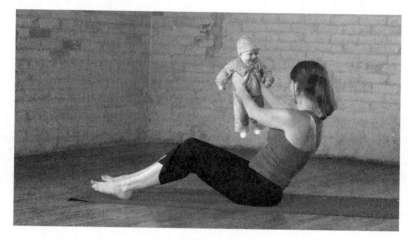

6. *Bicycle Crunches.* Start on the floor, lying on your back with your legs bent at the knees and hands behind your head. Lift your legs off the ground, but keep them bent at the knees. Slowly pull the left knee toward the right shoulder. Pull your head upward, bringing the left knee and right elbow together. Then return your leg to the starting point and switch legs. Repeat 25 times.

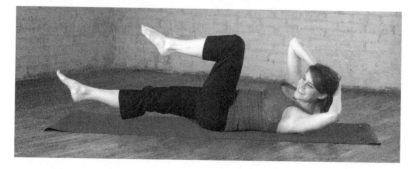

Since this exercise routine has a little cardio, I suggest that you end your workout with a cool-down and a stretch, to continue to enhance your flexibility.

Sanity Saver: Caffeine

Caffeine plays a central role in the lives of many new mothers. There are numerous ways to ingest this wonderful elixir, and I would say nearly every adult I know adheres to a preferred form. One of my best friends loves black tea, while another is a Diet Coke junkie. I know the preferred caffeinated beverage of each one of my closest friends. I know that two of my best childhood friends order skinny cinnamon dolce lattes, although one likes seven pumps of syrup while the other only likes two. It's a comforting treat and daily ritual for many moms.

While some will tell you to stay away from caffeine, medical researchers say that caffeine is okay while you are nursing and is recommended in moderation. For many, including me, it can be a sanity saver. I can't tell you how much I craved my morning ritual of a delicious cup of coffee during my first months as a new mom. I dealt with the baby all night long so my husband could sleep, since his life depended on it. (As a pilot, he needs to be awake!) Needless to say, I was pretty tired from taking care of all nighttime feedings.

My husband would bring the baby into our room in the morning so I could nurse in bed; then I'd let my daughter sleep on my chest from about 6 until 9 A.M. (which was such a beautiful time for me). I'd wake up and watch *The Today Show* while I nursed, and then we'd go downstairs. There, I had a soothing ritual of making myself coffee or a latte. I so looked forward to that cup of coffee, which somehow made me feel "adult" and in control. The baby was content and happy, having just been fed, so I'd sip my coffee and read a nice magazine or book that didn't require much brainpower.

My advice is to create a morning ritual that helps you get in a calm, peaceful, grateful mind-set to start your day. This may or may not include caffeine for you, but establish a ritual and set aside a time to get your day started right. Have something to look forward to that makes you feel put together (at least a little).

There is no doubt that too much caffeine can make your body feel stressed and your heart rate increase by stimulating the central nervous system. I also know there are many who believe that coffee has negative impacts on the adrenal glands. There may be some truth to this, but here are some of the numerous benefits of the polyphenols found in coffee and tea:

— Numerous studies indicate that people who drink coffee on a regular basis are up to 80 percent less likely to develop Parkinson's.[2]

— Caffeine is known to help treat asthma and headaches, which is why a dose of pain reliever such as Anacin or Excedrin contains up to 120 milligrams of it.

— Drinking at least two cups of coffee daily can translate to a 25 percent reduced risk of colon cancer, an 80 percent drop in liver cirrhosis risk, and nearly half the risk of gallstones.[3]

— Studies have found that coffee drinkers at midlife have a lower risk of dementia and Alzheimer's disease later in life compared to those drinking no or only little coffee. The lowest risk (a 65 percent decrease) was found among moderate coffee drinkers (consuming three to five cups of coffee a day).[4]

— Dr. Tomas DePaulis of Vanderbilt University is quoted as saying, "Overall, the research shows that coffee is far more healthful than it is harmful. For most people, very little bad comes from drinking it, but a lot of good."[5] When there is a legal compound out there that has all of these positive impacts when ingested in moderation *and* it helps sleep-deprived parents get through their days, then I say go for it! Enjoy!

So we know caffeine can give us a boost and has some health benefits, but what about nursing while drinking caffeine? Most experts agree that it is okay in moderation, and only one percent of the caffeine ingested gets into the breast milk. There are, of course, some babies with sensitive tummies who can't even tolerate that amount, but most should be just fine. The American Academy of Pediatrics has published that excessive caffeine (greater than 300 mg/day) can cause poor sleeping, irritability, and poor feeding in your baby and recommends limiting caffeine to one or two cups per day. Another important fact is that caffeine levels are found to be highest in breast milk one hour after drinking caffeinated beverages, so plan your drinking/feeding schedule accordingly.[6]

The La Leche League website quotes *The Womanly Art of Breast-feeding* for its recommended rule of thumb for nursing mothers, which is that five or fewer five-ounce cups of coffee should not cause a problem for most mothers and babies.

All of this research says to me that if you feel jittery and have negative physical effects from caffeine, then it's probably too much. Otherwise, simply enjoy. Trust your gut!

Affirmation for the Week

Raising a human being from birth is not for sissies. Motherhood might break me down, but I know it will also raise me up and make me stronger and happier than I could have imagined. My heart has expanded to new proportions, and I am continually in awe of my child's individuality and intelligence.

I will allow the motherhood experience to help me grow as a woman and improve my life overall. I will let my capacity to love expand, and I will follow my children's lead by living completely in the present

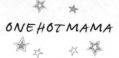

moment. I will strive to enjoy every fleeting minute with my baby and inhale his sweet smell before he grows up and won't let me snuggle. These days can be draining and may seem trivial, but they are precious and so influential on the rest of my child's life. I will live fully and love freely. I will remind myself daily what a blessing it is to be a mother, especially on those days that are particularly tough. I will also keep reminding myself that the difficult moments will pass, and I will be left with all the fun and beautiful memories that remain.

★❏★

Month 2 Workout Schedule

	Monday	Tuesday	Wednesday	Thursday	Friday	Saturday	Sunday
Week 5	30-minute walk or 20-minute jog	20 minutes strength	1-hour walk, 30-minute jog, or cardio class at gym	20 minutes strength	30-minute walk, 20-minute jog, or cardio class at gym	Yoga or Pilates class	Rest
Week 6	45-minute walk or 30-minute jog	20 minutes strength	1-hour walk, 30-minute jog, or cardio class at gym	20 minutes strength	30-minute walk, 20-minute jog, or cardio class at gym	Yoga or Pilates class	Rest
Week 7	45-minute walk or 30-minute jog	30 minutes strength	1-hour walk, 30-minute jog, or cardio class at gym	30 minutes strength	45-minute walk, 30-minute jog, or cardio class at gym	Yoga or Pilates class	Rest
Week 8	45-minute walk or 30-minute jog	30 minutes strength	1-hour walk, 30-minute jog, or cardio class at gym	30 minutes strength	45-minute walk, 30-minute jog, or cardio class at gym	Yoga or Pilates class	Rest

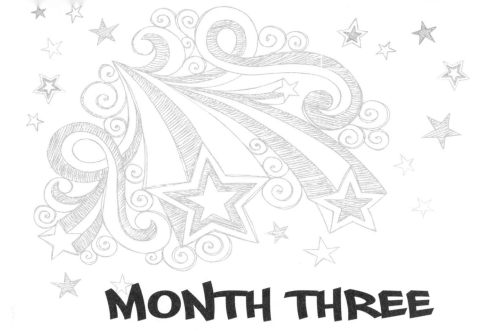

MONTH THREE

In this third and final month of getting yourself back after having a baby, you will be encouraged to dig deeper and do some soul searching to really know and understand yourself. Additionally, you will be inspired to strive for the right balance in your life—one that allows you to focus your time and energy on the things that mean the most to you while maintaining a lifestyle that suits your family. Getting your mama mojo flowing is the goal of Week 11, and Week 12 will leave you with the knowledge of how fabulous and strong you really are as you go on with your life as a mother.

★ ◻ ★

Soul Searching

"She who knows others is learned;
she who knows herself is wise."

—LAO-TZU, TAO TE CHING

Soul searching is the process of going within and contemplating your own beliefs about spirituality and the way you conduct your life. It's a form of introspection—of figuring out who you really are. Some people might not believe that motherhood is the best time to do this, but I don't think there is a better time. A love so deep and complex can open up our hearts to spirituality in an entirely new way. This love can also prompt us to evaluate the way we live and how we can do better. This is soul searching.

Experiencing the transformation of your own body to accommodate the development of a human being, followed by delivering that human being into the world, is transformational. Recognizing that two cells combined and kept dividing, each cell simply "knowing" what to do, can cause even the most non-spiritual person to contemplate the perfection and beauty of human life.

This week, I simply want to encourage you to look within. Many people go through a phase of introspection during their high school or college years, but now is a great opportunity to re-assess your life to make sure it is in alignment with who you really are and what you really want.

Knowing Yourself

Many of us have gone through our lives without taking the time for self-evaluation or getting to know ourselves on a deeper level. It is now time to reclaim who you are, what you believe, and what you want out of life. Many women I know have lost themselves to the point that their own preferences and desires have become edged out in the shuffle of their busy lives. Take this opportunity to look within and get in touch with your true self once again.

Your Beliefs and Convictions

What do you believe about people and life? Has a person or event made you question everything? Have you had a long-standing belief about something or someone that was changed in an instant? Or have your beliefs slowly changed over time?

The most interesting people we converse with are those with firm beliefs and convictions. While it's good to know who you are and what you believe in, I believe it is to your advantage to always remain open to new information. We can be very hard on politicians who "flip-flop," but I think that's the wisest thing people can do when they learn something new that causes them to see an issue in a different light.

For example, many people are anti-military because they believe that the military is a crew of violent people who join together to exert power and support all of our country's armed conflicts around the world. Before becoming intimately familiar with the military, I might have held that viewpoint. However, now that I am married to a military man (who is one of the most loving, nonviolent people I have ever met), I know that lumping everyone in the military into one group is unfair. Not only that, but I also know that many of my husband's colleagues care deeply about peace and using our armed forces to eventually create a better world. They believe that any violence created is in an effort toward the global greater good. These men and women are simply patriotic people who want to serve their country in a way that is virtuous and admirable.

The same goes for contentious issues such as global climate change, abortion, religion, and taxes. While you may believe that you understand all sides of an issue, do you really? Have you taken the time to research the issues that interest you to ensure that you know the unbiased truth? As a scientist by education, I place a lot of emphasis on doing research. I used to get most of my news from a select few sources, but now I realize that I need to branch out and read, listen to, and watch a variety of sources to get the entire picture.

What do you believe about God or universal love? Have you taken the time to meditate on what your beliefs truly are? Until I graduated from college, I simply did what my parents had done; I attended a Lutheran church and believed in what I was raised to believe. Then one day when I was in graduate school, I got curious and decided to explore religion and other ways people worshiped God. While living in downtown Minneapolis, I was in close proximity to countless churches and places of worship. I tried numerous denominations and realized that I enjoyed pieces of nearly every service I attended. I also came to understand that there was a common thread among them: love. It was such a great exercise for me, and it made me realize that my Lutheran roots were really beautiful but that I didn't need a Lutheran church to enjoy a close relationship with God.

Have you been to a place of worship lately? If not, why not? Would you enjoy it, or would it add something beneficial to your life? I do not think that churches, synagogues, and mosques are the only places to be close to God, but they do provide a sense of community and a ritual that can foster your spirituality in a beautiful way.

Have you read any spiritual books lately? There are countless authors out there who write in beautiful ways to inspire you to look within and connect with something bigger. Do you believe in angels? Do you believe in past lives? Do you believe in heaven and hell? It's hard to be sure about any of this, but learning and reading about these topics can help you shape your beliefs and satisfy some of your curiosity.

Your Strengths

Do you know what your strengths are, or have you even thought about them lately? If you know what they are, are you using them? Even as a stay-at-home mom, you can use your strengths in ways that make your world, and the world at large, a better place. You will feel a greater sense of satisfaction in life if you are using your God-given assets in some capacity.

There are many aptitude tests out there that you can use to hone in on your strengths. One that I took in college was the Myers-Briggs Type Indicator. It has to be given by a certified administer, but it is very comprehensive and can help you identify your strengths. The results of the test offer career areas that might help you use your natural gifts. My results indicated that my strengths were communication and empathy and that I should be in the field of teaching. So I went into science and engineering! Over ten years later, I finally opened my eyes to why I felt an underlying sense of dissatisfaction at work; I was not in a career that expressed my natural talents most fully.

If you still aren't exactly sure what your strengths are, ask a family member or a close friend. They might say things you hadn't thought of, such as that you are creative, funny, or organized. Your friends might focus on your traits that they most admire, which probably shine through for the rest of the world to see when you are at your best.

Understanding your strengths is also important to help you optimize your motherhood experience. Recognizing the situations that make you vulnerable can help you prop yourself up when necessary. Parenting from your strengths will inspire your children to grow up to more fully express themselves. I have a dear friend who is an amazing artist, and when I hear about the projects she is doing with her child, I think it is so cool; I wish I could think of those types of fun activities. She had her daughter painting as an infant! My children are exposed to great things but definitely not ultra-creative art projects—unless I get inspired by my friends or find an idea in a craft blog or magazine. Using your natural strengths both in and out of the home will bring you more joy in your daily life.

A great strength to have when trying to get your mind and body back after having a baby is self-discipline. Having discipline will help you get to bed early, make good food choices, and work out as often as possible. If self-discipline is not one of your strengths, just work a little harder in those areas. Self-discipline comes more naturally to some than others, but everyone can learn it.

Your Weaknesses

Knowing your weaknesses is nearly as important as knowing your strengths. Babies and small children introduce an element of stress that can amplify your weaknesses. Identifying the situations that cause you stress and discontent will help you minimize them. For example, if being late is a weakness of yours and it causes you stress to be running behind, you can make adjustments to your schedule to get places on time. Getting out the door with a baby can be a real challenge on some days, so it's important for all moms to develop a realistic schedule so they are not always running late.

Is your weakness a lack of self-esteem? In other words, do you need to feel wanted and popular to feel good about yourself? Do you require material objects to feel happy? Do you need attention from men to feel pretty? These are all common human weaknesses that can lead to some serious suffering, especially when you might be experiencing changes in your body and earning potential. Ideally, happiness and self-esteem come from within. Achieving this can take years of soul searching and getting to know yourself. Having babies and getting older can start taking a toll on what you perceive as your beauty, but as you go through your life, you will begin to realize that true beauty comes from your spirit—and the most beautiful people are those who radiate strength, kindness, and love.

Is your weakness food? Do you use food to comfort yourself to an extent that is unhealthy? It is human to use food for comfort, and it is not necessarily a bad thing—unless it becomes an addiction that causes you to gain unwanted weight or to remain at an unhealthy weight. Do you use food as a reward? Try to come up with non-food alternatives that are just as appealing, such as buying a new book or getting a pedicure. One square of dark chocolate can also do the trick if you really need an edible treat! If you are home with your baby and have easy access to food all day long, using unhealthy food to comfort yourself is a dangerous weakness. You can use a myriad of tools from this book and others to protect yourself against overeating.

One of my greatest weaknesses is being a serious night owl. I used to see this as a strength, but now that I have babies who wake before dawn, I absolutely have to get in bed at a decent hour or I can really suffer. Sometimes I find myself on an Internet searching, writing, or reading binge, and I just can't stop until my eyes are bulging and my body aches—usually during the wee hours of the morning. I regret my lack of self-discipline the next morning when I am up trying to feed children and get the oldest off to school bright and early. Getting ample sleep is crucial for my well-being in many ways, so I have finally bucked the night owl trend. One day, when my kids are all grown up, I might be able to express my natural night owl once again; but until then, I have decided I am better off with a full eight hours of sleep.

Your Conduct

Are you completely satisfied with the way you carry yourself and live your life? Would you want your daughter or son growing up to behave just like you? When I asked myself this question, I realized that in some ways, yes, but in some ways, definitely not.

As I have mentioned throughout this book, babies are watching and mentally capturing the way we behave so they can behave the same way. Think about the ways you conduct yourself daily that you are not exactly proud of, and then consider some more positive ways you can behave. Personally, I can have a bit of a temper and be defensive. I am sure my children have seen me staunchly defend myself on a comment or request made by my husband that I somehow took personally. Speaking of which, do you take things personally? We often take things personally that are in no way directed toward us or meant to harm us.

Do you talk negatively about the way you look? Do you want your daughters to mimic the way you treat your body? We can't be perfect all the time, but making an effort to be conscious of how we refer to ourselves can have a big influence on our children and how they will eventually regard themselves.

Do you talk to people in a fashion that is rude or abrupt? Do you treat others in a way that puts them at ease or on guard? The other day, a man came up to me in the grocery store and asked me if I knew where the beef broth was. I walked him to the section and pointed it out since I knew exactly where it was. I thought nothing of it, but my five-year-old daughter looked up at me and said, "Mommy, you're a nice person." It was one of the best compliments I have ever received. Trust me, I have also been the one stomping and ranting around the house because I can't find something or because I am frustrated. Those are moments I am not proud of, and I strive to minimize that crappy behavior because I know little eyes are watching my every move.

Your Attitude

I am a big believer that your enjoyment of life hinges, to a large degree, on your attitude. Have you taken the time to evaluate your attitude lately? Are you positive and optimistic or downright gloomy? There is no better time than the present to make an attitude adjustment. Unfortunate things are going to happen to you as a parent, such as getting pooped on, puked on, or peed on, or having your baby spit up all over his or her adorable, freshly washed outfit. You are going to have to miss out on fun events to stay home with a sick child. You might not be as free to spend money on your indulgences anymore. These things can feel restrictive and depressing—or you can see them as challenges to do more with less.

Use the obstacles associated with motherhood to push yourself to handle tough situations with grace and optimism. My mom is an extremely positive woman with a can-do attitude about everything. I am pretty sure that both my brother and I learned a lot of how we conduct our lives as adults from her. Of course, there are times when it's a struggle for anyone to have a positive attitude, and I also know that it comes more naturally to some than others. I can see the differences in the natures of my own children! However, when you are aware, you will learn to identify when you are having a crappy attitude and can make a conscious effort to turn it around!

Do you see the glass as half empty or half full? If you do not naturally see the world in a rosy hue, I want you to know that you can learn how. How do I know? Because I have seen a profound transformation in my husband over the past ten years of our marriage. My husband is a brilliant, left-brained fighter pilot who tends to have a bit of a negative attitude and a darker view of life. He does not naturally see the best in people. Over time, living with someone who so firmly believes in the power of a positive attitude has rubbed off on him. I can see how he has become more optimistic and upbeat about life in general. I think he also decided that he wanted to set a happier example for his children. Now this joyful attitude has become second nature to him. He is still the same wonderful, smart man—only better!

Our attitudes are largely made up of our habitual thought patterns. Pause to notice the initial thoughts that come into your mind during various situations. Does your thinking automatically go to the negative? Habitual thought patterns are difficult to break, but I am confident it can be done; I have seen it happen. For example, when someone is cold or rude to you, do you automatically think he or she must not like you or has something against you? It's easy to do. A more positive way of thinking is, *She must have a lot on her mind.* Don't take it personally, and move on.

My husband and I had an experience with this recently. A couple we know always seemed fairly cold to us and not really interested in talking to us or getting to know us. I tried to blow it off, but my husband took it personally; it really bugged him. The other night I was out with some women, and I heard them talking about this particular couple. They'd had terrible infertility problems and countless miscarriages—and here I was with a large belly and a baby on the hip. I instantly understood. This point came into clarity for me: Remain positive despite how people treat you, because you really have no idea what they are going through.

Finally, I want to share with you a few powerful statistics on how being optimistic and having a positive attitude can improve your life:

— Positive people have lower rates of depression as well as better psychological and physical well-being.[1]

— When people think positively, it enhances their immune systems, and they experience greater resistance to illnesses such as the common cold.[2]

— Positive people are shown to have healthier hearts and a reduced risk of death from cardiovascular disease.[3]

— Positive people generally have better coping skills during hardships and times of stress.[4]

— When people have a positive attitude, they experience significantly longer lives. In a study of nuns, those who regularly expressed positive emotions lived on average ten years longer.[5]

— Marriages between positive people have a significantly higher success rate. For example, research shows that marriages fare much better when a couple experiences a five-to-one ratio of positive to negative interactions. Conversely, when the ratio of positive to negative interactions starts to get closer to one to one, the marriage has a much higher chance of ending in divorce.[6]

— People who are positive report having more friends, and having more friends generally leads to greater happiness!

Creating Your Most Fabulous Future

Now that you are getting to know yourself better and are becoming more aware of your attitudes, motives, beliefs, strengths, and weaknesses, you can start to envision a future that displays your greatest talents and magnifies your spirit to the world.

Many go through life letting their futures simply "happen." I hope you are feeling empowered to take control of your life and create something even more special. Begin seeing each day as a gift, and get super excited about what the future holds. Imagine the joy of raising a baby into a happy, well-adjusted adult. See yourself for who you really are—a wonderful, kind, and talented woman who is going to set an amazing example for her children. In the final weeks, I will discuss visualization, so you can start seeing yourself morph into the best version of who you are.

Nourishment: Revisiting Your Overeating Pitfalls

Back in Week 3, you took a quiz to help you identify your overeating weaknesses. This week, about soul searching, seems like an ideal place to revisit overeating, which might be hindering your weight-loss efforts. Let's review the overeating pitfalls and explore a few coping methods for minimizing their impact on your weight-loss journey!

Unhealthy Habits

Habits are often very hard to break, which is why this pitfall can be one of the tougher ones to overcome. The first step in breaking a habit is to recognize that a particular act has become habitual. I have certainly had to overcome habitual eating habits that weren't so good, such as the ice cream habit I mentioned—or the chocolate croissant habit I developed during my third pregnancy. Once you recognize and believe that an eating habit is a problem, you can devise concrete steps to break it.

Second, you need to *want* to change the habit. If you firmly believe that your habit of eating Lucky Charms for breakfast is no longer serving you and you genuinely want to do something different, you will put the energy into finding an alternative that makes you happy but is much better for you. Maybe you will discover that whole grain blueberry waffles are so delicious that you don't miss the Lucky Charms!

This leads me to another important point. You need to find an acceptable alternative for the unhealthy food that brings you some level of satisfaction; otherwise you will be tempted to go right back to your bad habit. Find a healthy food that tastes just as good (or as close as possible, anyway) and will not take away from your quest for getting your ideal body back!

Finally, be as consistent as possible until your old bad habits are replaced with healthier ones. However, if you happen to fall off the wagon, take it easy on yourself, and reaffirm your commitment to healthier habits the next day.

Emotional Eating

Looking back at the quiz in Week 3, did you score high in the emotional eating section? This is a real issue for many women. Even those of us who don't always eat emotionally use food as a salve from time to time. The key is to identify when it's a problem.

How do you know when eating for comfort has become a problem? If you recognize any of the following behaviors in yourself, then emotional eating may pose challenges for you in your weight loss journey:

- When you are feeling overwhelmed and gloomy, you head for a fast-food fix or you pick up unhealthy food at the grocery store that you would normally avoid.

- On rough days, you eat more sugar, such as candy and chocolate—and it's a lot more than just a piece of candy or a square of chocolate.

- You crave fatty, rich foods when times are tough, and you indulge every time you get the craving.

- Your life has been particularly stressful or difficult in the past year (you've got a new baby, so chances are it has been!), which has caused you to hold on to all of your baby weight.

- You find yourself snacking throughout the day after a rough night up with the baby to try to make yourself feel better.

These are just a few indicators that emotional eating may be an issue for you to some degree. If food is something you use to make yourself feel better, try to discover foods that comfort you but have healthy ingredients. Take a step back before automatically reaching for food when you need comfort. Try some of the following alternatives when you're feeling overwhelmed, tired, or depressed: call a friend, take a bath, go for a walk, head to the gym, eat a delicious apple or one square of dark chocolate, get a skim-milk latte, arrange for a babysitter and escape to a bookstore or a spa, or take a nap.

Social Eating

The opportunities for social eating often decrease once motherhood arrives because social outings are generally less frequent. Their relative infrequency makes these outings more of a potential problem: We see eating at restaurants as a treat; therefore, we eat whatever we want and as much as we want. I have certainly been guilty of this!

Here are a few indications that social eating might be wreaking havoc on your efforts to lose baby pounds:

- You order things at restaurants that are completely uncharacteristic for you and unhealthy, because you feel like splurging.

- When you go out to dinner with your husband or friends, or when you go to parties, you get swept up in the festive atmosphere and end up impulsively eating really fattening foods.

- When you go out to socialize, you always end up having three or more sweet or alcoholic drinks.

- After a late night out, you crave pizza or nachos, just like when you were in college!

I want to stress that none of these behaviors is "bad," and eating fatty foods from time to time is part of being human! The problem occurs when you are trying to lose weight. You can undo a lot of progress with one particularly indulgent evening. New mothers generally don't have the opportunity to enjoy time out socializing with friends very often, but when you do get the chance, keep in mind the calorie counts of a few popular drinks and appetizers (so you can make better choices).

Calorie Counts of Popular Drinks and Appetizers

Drinks:[7]
Piña colada (6 oz.): 378 calories
Mojito (8 oz.): 214 calories
Cosmopolitan (4 oz.): 200 calories
Margarita (8 oz.): 280 calories
Long Island iced tea (8 oz.): 780 calories
Martini (2.5 oz.): 160 calories
Bloody Mary (5 oz.): 118 calories
Red wine (5 oz.): 120 calories
White wine (5 oz.): 120 calories
Beer (12 oz.): 150–198 calories
Light beer (12 oz.): 95–136 calories

Appetizers:[8]
Blooming onion/onion blossom: 1,552 calories, 83 g fat
Nachos (with chili and cheese): 1,680 calories, 108 g fat
Cheese fries: 2,100 calories, 150 g fat
Loaded potato skins: 1,000 calories, 100 g fat
Buffalo chicken wings (with ranch dressing): 900 calories, 60 g fat
Stuffed mushrooms: 300 calories, 19 g fat
Chicken lettuce wraps: 640 calories, 28 g fat
Shrimp cocktail: 120 calories, 1 g fat
Crab cakes: 300 calories, 16 g fat
Beef/chicken satay: 130 calories, 5 g fat
Edamame: 122 calories, 5 g fat

Mindless Eating

Moms with babies often suffer from two things: sleep deprivation and boredom. It's not that being home with a baby all day is necessarily boring, but if you are not working, your brain might not be stimulated as much as it would be otherwise. Boredom and exhaustion are both conditions that can make you ripe for eating mindlessly. When you are home, food is easy to access; without thinking, a tired mom can easily polish off a small bag of pita chips in search of a little pick-me-up. I know this because I have done it! Pita chips are a healthy food in moderation, but a whole bag is probably a bit too much!

Here are a few signs that you might be doing some mindless eating:

- You eat handfuls of snacks throughout the day because you're bored.

- You fill your plate, and without really paying attention to or enjoying your meal, you look down to find an empty plate.

- When you're tired, you grab a snack and then eat far more than you intended because you weren't paying attention.

- You frequently eat in front of the TV or while working on the computer.

You have the power to control your portion sizes. With a little awareness, this is one of the easiest overeating pitfalls to overcome. Mealtimes should be used for reconnecting with your family, and the food you eat should be enjoyed. When you take the time to focus only on your tablemates and how delicious your food tastes, you will feel satisfied with less. Slowing down is another way to ensure that you aren't mindlessly eating until you are stuffed. When you eat slowly and deliberately, you allow your body's natural "fullness triggers" to kick in.

Make it more difficult to grab snacks throughout the day so you will have to rely on your body's physiological triggers that you are hungry. For example, put your snack foods in a particular cupboard that is harder to get to so that you have to put in additional effort to retrieve them.

Be sure to have snack-sized bowls and plates available to help you serve yourself a proper portion. Over time, your body will adjust to an appropriate amount of food, which will start feeling like enough. Purchasing 100-calorie packages of snacks is useful to help you understand portion sizes. That's why I like to start my healthy-eating kicks with organic frozen meals, because they remind me of how much food I should be eating. Throughout my pregnancies, I forgot all about portion control and ate until I was full—and sometimes stuffed—because I was so hungry. After the babies were born, when I was trying to get my body back in shape, I needed to be reminded about how much food constitutes a 400-calorie meal.

Remember, this weight loss plan is not about deprivation; it's about really enjoying the food you eat and consuming the amount your body needs to be healthy. It is also important to be aware while you eat so that you are in touch with your body's natural mechanisms for letting you know it has had enough. It is not pleasant to feel overstuffed and bloated!

Lack of Motivation to Exercise

Exercising is a habit, and it can become such an important part of your daily routine that you will miss it if you don't do it. However, I know there are many out there who never get to the point of enjoying exercise. My mom tries to exercise, begrudgingly, but she has never loved it or been eager to get to the gym. We all have those days!

If you still don't feel like exercise is enjoyable or fun, here are a few of the most compelling reasons to head outside and exercise or go to the gym (in addition to the fact that you will be burning calories!):

- You are reducing your risk of osteoporosis, heart disease, and countless other health problems.

- You will have more self-confidence.

- Buying clothes will be more fun when you are fit and things fit better.

- You will want to have sex more often.

- You will have more energy.

- The more muscle you have, the more calories your body will burn at rest.

- You will sleep better.

Convinced? Over time, working out will truly become part of your life; you will want and need it, and you will miss it on the days you are too busy to fit it in. Eventually you will start to notice the effects that exercise has on your mind and body—and hopefully, you will determine that the discomfort and trouble are completely worth it.

On the days you are truly too exhausted to go to the gym, go for a walk. Walking is the perfect exercise when you are tired or unmotivated because you literally just have to go outside and put one foot in front of the other. After a while, your pace will pick up, and you will start to feel invigorated.

Here are a few other ideas to motivate you to get outside or to the gym for a good workout: buy yourself a cute new workout outfit, load your iPod or other MP3 player with some fun and interesting podcasts to listen to while walking or jogging, purchase or check out an unusual or fun-looking workout video (think belly dancing), or call a friend and schedule a workout date.

Fitness: Exercising for Inner Peace

Working out becomes a form of spirituality for many, especially those who exercise out in nature. Being outside helps these people connect with the natural world. Bikers, surfers, runners, and hikers report feeling connected to God or a higher spirit while out sweating in nature's beauty. I have experienced this type of euphoria when my body is doing a physical activity but my head is in a nearly meditative state. Many even pray or ponder the bigger spiritual issues of life while doing outdoor sports.

The act of being completely focused on what you are doing out of necessity is also a key component of inner peace. Rock climbing or doing something that requires your absolute attention can bring you a sense of purpose and calm. When you are doing a mindless exercise, on the other hand, your brain is allowed to roam freely. Sometimes when I am running, my brain jumps from topic to topic until I have thought about everything that needs a little consideration in my life. Afterward, I am calmer and my brain is available to completely focus on the task at hand.

Of course, yoga is what comes to mind as a form of exercise for achieving inner peace. Yoga is, in itself, a form of spirituality and can no doubt bring an amazing sense of inner peace. Those who have practiced yoga long enough will tell you that it has brought them a newfound sense of body awareness, inner stillness, and overall well-being. Once the physical act of yoga becomes part of your routine, the mystical aspect can enhance your spiritual life and help you feel more connected with God.

Can you incorporate at least one "spiritual" workout this week? Week 9's workout schedule has multiple opportunities for incorporating exercises that make you feel spiritually connected. Take a restorative yoga class, go for a walk, or run on a gorgeous nature trail. Pay attention and see if you can experience something spiritual during many of your week's workouts.

Week 9 Workout Schedule

Monday	Tuesday	Wednesday	Thursday	Friday	Saturday	Sunday
45-minute walk or 30-minute jog	30 minutes strength	1-hour walk, 40-minute jog, or cardio class at gym	30 minutes strength	45-minute walk, 30-minute jog, or cardio class at gym	Yoga or Pilates class	Rest

Spiritual Yoga Strengthener

Do the first three positions on your right side, and then repeat all three on the left side. Do the entire sequence of six exercises three times. Warm up with some deep breathing or with the gentle yoga routine outlined in Week 1.

1. *Warrior II Pose (Virabhadrasana II).* Place your feet about four feet apart, turning your right foot so the toes point toward the front of your mat. Next, turn your left foot inward 30 degrees. Raise your arms parallel to the floor, shoulder height, with your palms facing down. Bend your right knee to a 90-degree angle, tucking in your tailbone and keeping your core tight. Hold for five slow breaths. Go from Warrior II directly into the next pose, Reverse Warrior II.

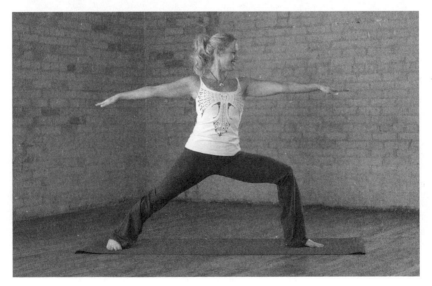

2. *Reverse Warrior II Pose.* From the Warrior II Pose with your right knee bent, bring your left hand down to rest on your left leg, which is still straight. Inhale as you reach your right arm up toward the ceiling. As you breathe, reach and stretch your arm even further. Be sure to keep your right knee bent, pressing into your feet with your legs strong. Sink your hips down toward the floor, and relax your shoulders. Hold for five breaths or up to a minute. To release, inhale while lowering your arms parallel to the floor, coming back into Warrior II.

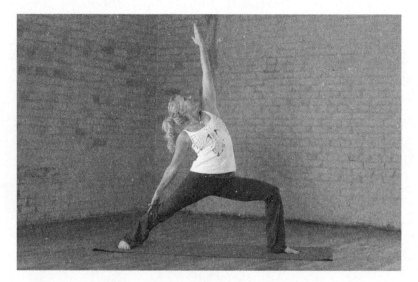

3. *Triangle Pose (Utthita Trikonasana).* Straighten both legs and raise your arms parallel to the floor, actively reaching out to the sides with your palms down. Turn your right foot to the right at a 90-degree angle and your left foot in slightly. Exhale and extend your torso directly out over your right leg, bending from your waist. Let your right hand drop to rest on your right shin or ankle, and then stretch your left arm toward the ceiling. Gaze forward to turn gently upward. Work to keep your body in alignment, imagining that you are pressed between two panes of glass. Hold the pose for five breaths or for a minute, and inhale as you come up.

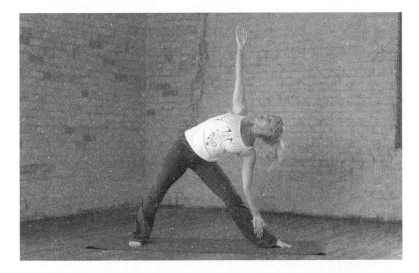

Now repeat these three poses on the left side before moving on to Tree Pose.

4. *Tree Pose (Vrksasana)*. From a standing position (Mountain Pose), shift your weight onto your left foot. Bend your right knee, and reach down with your right hand and clasp your right ankle. Lift your right foot up, and place the sole of your foot against your inner calf, thigh, or groin, depending on your flexibility and balance. Try to keep your hips even and neutral. Slowly lift your arms up above your head. Fix your gaze on a fixed object in front of you, and hold for five breaths or up to a minute on each leg.

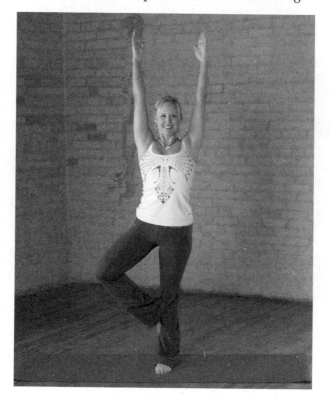

5. *Downward Dog (Adho Mukha Svanasana).* Start on the floor on your hands and knees, and then straighten your knees during an exhalation. Lift your hips toward the ceiling and keep your neck neutral. Slowly bend and straighten your knees while stretching your calf muscles one at a time to loosen them up. Slowly straighten your legs and press your heels toward the floor. Breathe deeply and relax into the pose for up to a minute.

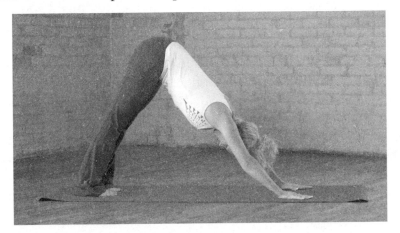

6. *Child's Pose (Balasana).* Start by sitting on your heels with your knees about as wide as your hips. Lay your body down between your legs with your arms outstretched in front of you or down along your legs with your palms up. Rest in this position for at least a minute.

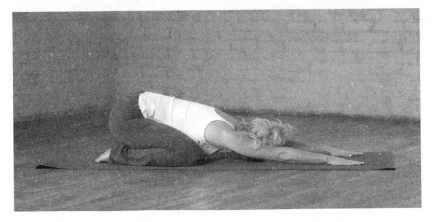

Sanity Saver: Time Alone

When you become a mother, weeks and days can go by without more than a few minutes to yourself. When our children are newborns, we might get a little extra time alone, but oftentimes we need to catch up on rest or housework during those moments.

Regardless of your children's ages, I want to challenge you to take time to do something completely alone. You might want to indulge in one of your guilty pleasures or maybe hang out at a coffee shop and read an engrossing book or the newspaper. Go for a hike on a beautiful trail, all by yourself.

Solitude is important for maintaining a sense of inner peace. I think that's why I love taking baths. I can go into the bathroom and be completely alone for a little while. That's also why I love my time in the morning before my family wakes. Feel a sense of gratitude for the silent and peaceful moments, as well as for the times when your home is full of sounds and laughter. If you have a partner or have a family member nearby, depend on them to watch the baby for an hour or two so you can get away and be alone.

The Importance of Solitude

You can actually hear your deepest needs and desires when it's quiet. In solitude, you can center your mind and connect with a higher power. How can you expect to know your deepest desires, dreams, and needs if you don't take time to listen to your soul? It is during the quiet moments when the visions we have for ourselves become more clear.

Here are a few ways to have some quiet time, all alone:

— Go away on an overnight retreat. There are many religious, meditation, writing, and yoga retreats where you will be afforded time alone for silence and solitude. You might want to wait until your baby is a bit older, but you can always start planning and dreaming.

— Wake up early for silence, prayer, and meditation.

— When your partner gets home in the evening, head to the library and read magazines and pick out a few new books.

— Do something athletic on your own, such as a hike, bike ride, or run.

— Stay in a hotel for a night or two alone. My husband gave me the gift of a night at a beautiful hotel on the ocean for Mother's Day when my oldest child was one. I read, wrote, sipped wine, and slept for 12 hours. I arrived back home feeling completely refreshed and rejuvenated. I made sure my husband could see how recharged and happy I was, so this was a gift he knew to give me every year.

— Spend a few hours, or even a day, at home alone. Pick up and organize your house so that it feels completely peaceful and orderly; then lie around and read, journal, nap, or simply revel in the solitude.

— Go out and have a cup of coffee or glass of wine by yourself. It's empowering to have the confidence to sit somewhere by yourself and enjoy a drink. Bring a book or magazine to enjoy.

Affirmation for the Week

Knowing and understanding myself is an important step in self-actualization and living my life to its highest potential. I am now more aware of my strengths and weaknesses so I can tailor my life in a way that allows me to use my strengths for my greatest good while minimizing the complications that my weaknesses can potentially bring to my life. Soul searching is helping me know and understand myself, to enhance my spirituality and become a more deeply divine and connected woman.

★❑★

The Constant Quest for Balance

"Women need real moments of solitude and self-reflection to balance out how much of ourselves we give away."

— BARBARA DE ANGELIS

In working with hundreds of moms, there is one thing I know for sure: We all crave balanced lives with enough time for those things we want and need to be happy. Most of us strive to maintain a sense of equilibrium in our lives, with success often coming in waves.

There are days and even weeks when I feel like my life has struck a perfect balance. During those times, I work two full days a week, spend lots of focused and loving time with my kids, have time alone with my husband, wake up early to meditate and pray, talk to my faraway family, have lunch or coffee with girlfriends, exercise six days a week, make healthy meals, sleep at least seven hours a night, and feel a sense of overwhelming joy and well-being.

But . . . then a work deadline comes along and things begin to come a bit unraveled in my home. Life just starts getting out of whack when I am super busy, and I feel unbalanced. Suddenly, I don't make it to the gym for a few days, the refrigerator becomes empty, laundry piles up, and our home life becomes a bit disheveled. Our meals go from decent, homemade ones to takeout and quickly cooked ones. My kids notice because they spend more time with a babysitter, so when I am with them, they adhere themselves to my side. The toddler clings to my leg, and my mommy guilt kicks in strongly because I am clearly not spending enough time with my precious children.

Take a look at the following list of items. Number them 1 through 13 in the "Your Priority" column; rank them in order of importance to you, with 1 being the most important thing in your life. In the second column, number the items in order of how much time you spend on them, with 1 being the most time.

	Your Priority	Your Reality
Career climbing		
Time with children		
Clean and orderly house		
Exercising		
Financial security		
Relationship with spouse		
Relationships with friends		
Relationships with parents/siblings		
Inner peace/meditation		
Spirituality/God		
Creative endeavors		
Eating healthy		
Watching TV		

How do your numbers match up? I have found, and research has proven, that dissatisfaction in life comes when people are not living in alignment with their priorities. This means that if you value your relationship with God and inner peace but spend five minutes a day meditating and two hours watching TV, then you are not in alignment. Or if your relationship with your husband ranks in your top three but the time and effort you spend on him are substantially lower, then something needs to change. You might argue that you have to work and it's not a choice, which I understand and respect. Full-time jobs tend to throw a few things out of whack, such as exercising and creative endeavors. However, you can make sacrifices and rearrange a few things in your life to create more time for the things that really bring you joy.

Some people believe that life is drudgery, and they just try to "get through" each day. In my opinion, this disrespects the opportunity and blessing of experiencing life on earth! We are here to live and experience feeling, meaning, and joy to the very fullest. If your life, in its current configuration, is not bringing you that joy, then things should be changed.

Dr. Wayne Dyer always says, "Feeling good is feeling God." He is not talking about the temporary good feelings after doing something like drugs, which cause long-term harm to your life and body. He is talking about feeling and loving the joys and pleasures that life can bring. An example is snuggling with a freshly bathed baby (who is giving off that special baby smell), who looks up to you and gives you a big, toothless grin. That is a simple but absolutely precious and pure bit of bliss.

If you really think about your day, the opportunities to experience and appreciate joy are endless: the colorful sunrise, your cozy bed, cuddling with your children, a hot cup of coffee or tea, your favorite breakfast, the beauty of the trees on a walk or jog, an engaging conversation with a stranger, a call from your mom or a best friend, a hug from your spouse, feeling centered after a little prayer or meditation, or a good song on the radio on your drive to work. I could go on and on! Notice these wonderful little things, and life will seem so much more pleasant and enjoyable.

In the next sections, I will cover some things that women struggle to balance every day. I will offer a few suggestions for how we can strive to maintain the balance that feels best to each of us.

Working vs. Staying Home with Family

There is no doubt in my mind that this is one of the most difficult decisions most mothers struggle with. I addressed working versus staying home in Week 2 in regard to money, but this week, I am going to talk about it in terms of living a balanced, happy life. As I have alluded to, there are many women who are certain they want to be home with their babies. Their decision is easy, although the financial sacrifices required to make that happen may be difficult. Others know without a doubt that they want to work full-time and continue on their career paths.

There are significant benefits and drawbacks to every situation related to working or staying home. Here are a few questions for you: Do you feel satisfied with whatever situation you are in right now? If not, what is at the core of your dissatisfaction? Is there a way you can work and still achieve the life balance that feels right to you? Are you able to work full-time and still give yourself, your body, your health, your spouse, and your children the love and attention they require? If you stay home full-time, do you feel fulfilled and challenged, or do you feel lonely and bored?

This aspect of your life can be terribly difficult to balance, but the more you thoughtfully weigh your options and listen to your heart, the better decisions you will make for you and your family. My cousin didn't work while her children were babies and toddlers. She loved her days of being home with the kids, going to a gym that had childcare, and feeling like she had her home life very under control. As her children grew up, she eventually felt it was time to go back to her career as a teacher, and so she did. At the end of the eight-hour workday, she devoted herself and the remainder of her time to her three children. She felt this was necessary because her husband traveled for his job and was away at least a week or two each month. Taking time for herself and exercising went completely by the wayside. In this type of situation, many women start to gain weight and feel like they are losing themselves. My cousin eventually realized that her life was out of balance, and she is now taking concrete steps to exercise five days a week and make herself and her health a priority.

Financial Security vs. Time to Enjoy Life

On a similar note, many of us, and our husbands for that matter, continue to work long hours at stressful jobs because we value a sense of financial security and the finer things that money can bring. Many of us have to keep our long-hour jobs to provide our families with health care. I know there are countless reasons to keep draining jobs, whether it's to simply put food on the table or whether it's to afford the payments on your 4,000-square-foot house or new car.

It is not my intention to judge; I simply hope to get you to think critically and deeply about what we exchange for material objects. If you are going to sacrifice time with your children and husband, friendships, time alone, exercising, or whatever it might be, then I want you to be very certain it's the right decision for you.

I have worked full-time hours while raising children, so I know it's difficult, no matter what anyone says. While working was great, and I enjoyed both the challenges and the abundant money in my checking account, I felt like the rest of my life was completely unbalanced. All I wanted at the end of a long day was to snuggle with my kids, so taking additional time away to go to the gym or go for a run made me seethe in guilt. Many working moms have the discipline to wake up at 4:30 A.M. to exercise, but that just doesn't sound enjoyable to me. I greatly admire those who can do it!

While I was working full-time, cooking meals and ensuring our home had ample food and supplies even felt like a lot of work. Many women have husbands who are able to support them more in managing the household, which makes working full-time much more doable. My husband is in the military, where the hours are insane and inflexible. I had to do it all, and it is a lot of work, as any military spouse, single mother, or person married to a traveling professional can attest. Balance under these circumstances can be even more challenging.

Sit quietly and envision the work-life balance that would allow you the time for all the things that bring you the most pleasure and satisfaction in life. What are you willing to sacrifice, materially, to achieve that balance? Can you work part-time? Do you desire a job outside the home for your greatest joy? How can you balance a job with your home life and the things that bring you joy?

You have the power to create the ideal situation for yourself. Become clear as to what your ideal balance is, and then take concrete steps to make it happen. I know you can do it, and you will be much happier for living in alignment with your priorities!

Society's Ideal vs. Your True Self

Many women feel pressure to measure up to certain standards, whether it's the way your home is decorated, the way you dress, the meals you cook, the achievements of your children, or the condition of your body. I have lived all over the United States and have discovered that different communities and circles of women value different things. Mothers often feel a sense of pressure to do it all and be it all. Many of us find ourselves morphing into people we don't recognize, with priorities we aren't even sure are our own.

In many military circles, women pride themselves in being exceptionally talented homemakers. It can be difficult to carry on careers with the continual moving, so energy is thrown into decorating, crafting, cooking, or homeschooling. It's incredible what many of these women are capable of! There are women, though, like me, for whom these things are not particularly enjoyable and don't come naturally; we might feel inauthentic spending substantial amounts of time on crafts or things done merely to fit in.

Have you ever felt stressed just getting ready for a girls' night out because everyone else always dresses so fashionably and looks so put together that it creates a sense of pressure for you? I have. This is silly, and it takes away from the fun of cutting loose with good friends. Your girlfriends love you for who you are (or they should!) and appreciate your style, whatever it is. If you couldn't care less about designer clothes, then wear what feels good and flattering to you. Enjoy the process of making yourself look pretty rather than viewing it as a competition to look like someone else's ideal!

Perfectionism is a dangerous pursuit for all women, but for mothers in particular. You can completely unbalance your life in the pursuit of something that just doesn't exist. Oftentimes perfectionism is a mask for one's underlying unhappiness in life or with oneself. Sometimes it's a vestige of childhood. Does perfectionism cause any trouble for you? If so, what are some ways you can let go and live with peace and ease?

Is there any part of your life that feels inauthentic? Have you done things to fit in to society's ideal, even if it doesn't feel right or brings you stress? Are you doing something or acting in a way to please others, even if it causes you stress or disharmony? What does the real you like doing? What brings you pleasure? I encourage you to live and spend your time doing things that fit into *your* ideal, not your girlfriends' ideal or the ideal of society at large. Be yourself!

Clean-Enough House vs. Constantly Cleaning

Any woman with children knows that you can clean for hours a day and your house will still not be perfect. Living creates messes and dirt, and it's simply a losing battle if you are in pursuit of sterile perfection.

Find the balance that works for you. Pick up just once a day or at certain intervals rather than bending over constantly. Clean on a schedule so you don't have to think about it until it's time to actually do it. And as I've said before, you might need to lower your standards just a bit. Life is too short and precious to clean for hours a day. Think of it this way: Your children will have better immune systems if their surroundings aren't too sterile!

On the flip side, living in disorder and filth is not healthy for anyone, physically or mentally. You do want a sense of peace when you enter your home, not pure chaos or stress at the messiness. If you get anxious every time you walk into your house, then maybe you need to put a little more time into de-cluttering, organizing, and neatening up. Finding the balance that gives you a sense of comfort and calm in your home (without being a raving, cleaning lunatic) is what we are striving for!

Fit Enough vs. Exercising Endlessly

Even though this book is related to eating well and achieving your ideal weight, I still want to encourage you to think about your ideal weight and body and the time and effort you would have to put in to achieve it. I am all about exercising for an hour on most days, but if you are doing a lot more than that because you want to weigh 120 pounds, like you did in high school, perhaps you should think about your reasoning. Maybe your new "happy weight" is something a little higher than when you were 20 years old—and that's okay.

I have seen women become obsessed with getting skinny and working out. If you exercise to the point of utter exhaustion every day, then you are overworking your muscles and potentially causing more harm than good. Your workouts should include days that push you to your limits, combined with enjoyable yoga classes and easy jogs with your stroller. Your muscles have to recover from exertion, and the last thing you want to do is tear your body down and continually over-train to the point of exhaustion. No new mom needs that kind of pressure or extra strain!

You should definitely make exercising a priority in your life, but it has to be balanced with everything else you've got going on. Putting your baby in the stroller for 45 minutes is beneficial for both of you. Taking your children to the gym's childcare so you can fit in a spinning class once or twice a week is also just fine for your kids. Balancing exercising with all of the other demands of motherhood can be quite challenging at times, but if you want to look and feel your most fabulous, then you just have to fit it in. You will find the balance where you work out enough to maintain a healthy weight and look great without pushing yourself to the point of exhaustion. Recall all the reasons we exercise—to have boundless energy, set a great example for our children, feel sexy, look fit, and be confident. Remember that a balanced life includes fitness, but fitness and your body shape and size shouldn't consume you.

Time with Children vs. Time to Ourselves

It is a basic tenet of my life and writing that moms need time to themselves for rest, creativity, exercise, meditation, or whatever they value. Every woman's needs are different, but I want you to ask yourself if you get enough time to pursue your dreams and care for your mental and physical health.

I wholeheartedly believe that balanced moms are happy moms. If you feel as though you are happiest when devoting all of your waking hours to your children, then that is wonderful. Many of us feel ourselves slipping away when the scales are tipped that far in our children's favor. I am not proposing that you ignore your children all day so you can work on your current project, because that's not being a good mom either. Seek the balance of giving your children completely focused attention when you are spending time with them so they know how much you adore them—but also having time for outside interests, creative outlets, and intellectual activities. It's healthy for children to see that there are times when you are not dedicated to being their full-time playmate, and they need to entertain themselves a bit. It is also great for children to see their mothers living well-rounded, balanced, and happy lives.

Time with Children vs. Time with Our Partners

Raising babies and children can be so consuming that our partners inadvertently become second fiddle in our lives. Considering that a healthy and strong marriage is one foundation for a nurturing and loving home, this cornerstone relationship should be prioritized as much as possible. Of course, caring for the immediate needs of your children often takes priority, but carving out one-on-one time with your spouse is absolutely essential if you want your marriage to weather parenthood.

I don't want to imply that this is easy, because it's not. In fact, after ten years of marriage, my husband and I continually have to recommit to balancing our lives to include more time together, especially after the arrival of our surprise third baby! The effort is worth it. You and your partner will remain happier in your relationship, which will lead to greater life satisfaction.

At times, you might even have to sacrifice in other areas to ensure adequate time is dedicated to nurturing this relationship. Let's say you haven't worked out in a week, you have a huge deadline, and you have a sick baby. How do you balance everything and not lose your mind? Here's what I suggest for a balanced, best-case evening in this situation: Work a little late to get your deadline under control (while the baby is snuggled up resting), and then have the healthiest possible dinner delivered or have your partner pick it up on his way home. Have dinner with your family, and try to catch up as much as you can with your man. Snuggle the sick child, and put all the children to bed as early as possible. Then, put in a 30-minute exercise video, or even better, do a yoga workout.

After working out, take a hot bath, and then have your husband meet you for a glass of wine and a half-hour of talking and reconnecting. Watch your favorite TV show, then head to bed at 10 P.M. to either pass out or have a quickie. Try to convince your husband to give you a massage—you are in desperate need! Do not go to sleep any later than 11 P.M. to ensure that you get enough sleep to handle the stress of your deadline. Who knows? You might get awakened during the night by the wee one, but try to relax and enjoy quiet time during the feeding. Wait a good three to four minutes before running into the baby's room during a nighttime cry; hopefully the baby will fall back asleep! Or if your husband is willing, let him get up with the baby so you can sleep with earplugs. If he does this for you, be sure to show your appreciation with your positive energy and flirty smiles the next day.

Every day will bring new challenges to deal with, but take every opportunity to balance the multitude of things in your life with this key relationship. Go for a jog together after work, or put the baby in a baby backpack and go for a quick hike. Activities that let you get some exercise or do something creative or spiritual while enjoying your partner are an added bonus for balance!

Nourishment: Balancing Taste with Time and Health When Cooking

There is a widely held belief that you can't have it all, especially when it comes to food. Thankfully, this belief is completely untrue. You can have meals that are absolutely delicious and enjoyable but don't take hours to prepare—and will nourish your body. Elaborate, gourmet recipes have their time and place, but on a daily basis, they usually take too long.

So, how can you feed your family well without spending too much time and energy? Keep things simple, with uncomplicated recipes that require only a few ingredients. Broiled salmon with brown rice and steamed vegetables takes literally 20 minutes to prepare. If you use good spices and get the timing of everything right, this meal will undoubtedly be yummy.

In addition, develop a base of standby recipes, and keep your pantry stocked with the basic ingredients for them. There are a few recipes I have made so many times that I have them completely memorized and try to improve on them a little each time. They are generally super easy and well-loved by my husband and kids alike.

Learn how to cook meat and vegetables properly. There are many vegetables that I assumed I didn't like because I had only been exposed to soggy, canned versions as a child growing up in South Dakota. When I experienced fresh artichokes, asparagus, and various greens, prepared in delectable ways as an adult in California, I was absolutely floored by how delicious they were! I have slowly learned the right way to cook these things myself and continually try to prepare new and exciting vegetables. Cooking strange vegetables can be intimidating, but the reward of eating well-prepared, fresh veggies is worth it.

The same thing goes for lean meats. Overcooking lean meat, such as chicken or pork, is an easy mistake to make and will cause the meat to become dry and chewy. Do a little research on your computer or with a good cookbook, such as *Joy of Cooking* or *Martha Stewart's Cooking School*. With a little practice, you, too, can make meals with lean meats and lots of vegetables that taste incredibly good.

Pasta is another easy, quick meal. Pasta gets a bad rap from people watching their weight, but I disagree. Of course, portion control is the key. But whole wheat pasta or pasta cooked al dente (not too soft) is actually good for you. You can add all kinds of spices, meats, and vegetables for a really well-rounded meal. Another great perk of pasta is that kids love it. My children are always happy to eat pretty much any type of pasta! Getting creative with stir-fried dishes is also a good idea. Start with some cut-up meat, add vegetables, and serve with brown rice! The key to making stir-fry taste great is making delicious sauces that don't add too many calories but lots of flavor.

You may only have an infant right now, so this isn't an issue . . . yet. I advise you to do everything in your power to have your children, starting at toddler age, eat whatever you make for dinner. If they like the things separated or the sauce on the side, fine. But to keep meals easy and balanced, you should never, ever start becoming a line-order cook, preparing special items to suit your child's tastes. My husband helped me become strong in this area because, like many mothers, I have just wanted my children to eat enough food at times! If you expose your children to a variety of foods and get them to try at least one bite of everything, you are doing them a huge favor in the long run. They will learn to eat what they are served, and if they don't, they might be a little hungry. Never force your children to eat anything, but encourage them to try things and never let them dictate what they want in lieu of what's being served. Eventually, they will eat at least some of what you serve them, and your life will be easier.

Another great tip for helping your children learn how to be healthy eaters is to let them have fruit or yogurt for desert. We didn't learn this trick with our first child, who is a sugar lover and somewhat picky to this day. We did, however, convince her siblings that fruit and yogurt were treats to be savored as dessert, and they believe it wholeheartedly. I learned this trick from my sister-in-law, who let her daughters have a yogurt tube or pieces of pineapple as "dessert" after dinner. My nieces eat fruit as though it's the best treat they could possibly be offered!

Fitness: A Balanced Fitness Lifestyle

Ideally, exercising will simply become a well-loved part of your daily life. Any balanced lifestyle includes some form of fitness, including workouts that are effective as well as fun. The most fit and healthy women do a wide variety of exercises to create the most balanced physique possible. That's why my weekly workouts include a mix of cardio, strength, and flexibility or balance workouts, such as yoga. If you only do cardio, you will definitely achieve cardiovascular fitness and burn calories. However, building muscles will help your body burn more calories at rest; therefore, increased strength will complement your cardiovascular fitness. Yoga is the ultimate balancing exercise, working to improve your literal and emotional balance while evenly stretching and toning your body. Pilates is another wonderful exercise for balanced fitness. To elaborate on why you will be better off if you do a mix of cardio, strength, and stretching, I have included a little information on the benefits of each.

Cardio

Simply put, you must get your heart rate up if you want to lose weight. It is the most important component of your exercise program. Cardio workouts burn the most calories and really benefit your heart. You need to sweat and breathe hard a few times each week to get in the best shape! It is easy to increase the rate at which you burn calories during cardio exercise by quickening your pace slightly, going up hills, or trying something completely different and new that challenges your muscles. Higher-impact exercises that involve running and jumping will be more effective, more quickly, than lower-impact activities. You can achieve a certain level of cardio fitness by walking alone, but you would really benefit from adding exercises that use both your upper and lower body, such as cross-country skiing and high-intensity aerobics classes.

The key to a good cardio workout is to make sure you are sweating and really getting your heart pumping. It can feel so rejuvenating and therapeutic to work up a good sweat! The best cardio exercises include running, biking, hiking, spinning classes, high-impact aerobics, and plyometric exercises (such as jumping and burpees).

Weight-bearing exercises are crucial for helping women build bone and prevent osteoporosis later in life. Activities such as running, dancing, and even brisk walking will help. Researchers have discovered two factors that should be present to realize the best bone fortification: Higher-strain magnitude and repeated strain (such as running) equaled better bone fortification.[1]

Strength

A balanced fitness routine always includes some form of strength exercise. If going to the gym and lifting weights doesn't appeal to you, don't fear. There are countless other types of workouts that can strengthen your muscles effectively, such as yoga; Pilates; and weight-bearing strength exercises such as push-ups, squats, and dips. You really only need two or three strength workouts each week to have an effect, and they don't have to take too long!

Cardio comes easily for me because I enjoy it, but working on my strength does not. That is why I have developed this list of reasons—to convince both you and me, as to why we should include strength training as a key component of our fitness routines:

1. *Strength training improves and restores bone density.* Similar to weight-bearing exercises, strength training is important for helping you fortify your bones, to prevent osteoporosis.

2. *Stronger muscles help you prevent injury.* The stronger you are, the less likely you are to injure yourself while running or even

while just playing around with your children or rearranging your living room!

3. *Having more lean muscle mass increases your metabolism.* Yes, you read this right! The more muscle you have, the more calories you will burn while at rest. This is my favorite!

4. *Strength exercises slow your aging rate.* As we age, we naturally start to lose muscle mass, and our metabolisms slow down, as well. It's essential to keep our muscles toned and strong for many reasons, but one of the most important is to maintain a healthy metabolism rate as we get older.

5. *Strength training helps you look more toned and defined.* There is no doubt that you will look more toned by doing cardio, but strength exercises can take your body to a whole new level of fitness and definition. Some women worry that lifting weights or any form of strength exercise will bulk them up, but this is usually impossible because women don't produce enough testosterone for that. If this concerns you, do low- or no-weight strength exercises with higher repetitions.

Flexibility and Balance

Have you ever noticed a woman who has phenomenal posture; holds her head high; and has a long, lean, balanced look? Her graceful stature and dignified posture make her exude confidence! More often than not, women like this practice yoga or dance. Daily stretching and regular yoga are key components of feeling limber and lovely.

Many moms suffer from back and shoulder pain caused by nursing babies and lugging little ones around. Sometimes I worry that my spine is going to be permanently curved toward the left because I am always carrying a baby or child on my left hip. The thing that always brings both my mind and body back into balance is yoga. The twists and folding poses release a lot of tension along my spine and shoulders. I can walk into a yoga class with a desperate desire for a massage and leave having no need at all. Regular yoga also helps women have better posture and flexibility.

Why is flexibility important? A full range of motion, produced by flexible joints, is crucial for feeling fabulous. Flexibility actually increases blood flow to your muscles, speeding repair and recovery. Flexibility also reduces the potential for injury and can enhance your athletic performance. Have you ever experienced tight, knotted-up muscles? I have, and there is nothing better than a yoga class and a hot bath to soothe your painful muscles and induce complete relief.

Why is balance important? Let me count the ways! Believe it or not, a sedentary lifestyle can cause your balance to decrease dramatically. Loss of stability and balance is something we should all strive to prevent by exercising. Yoga offers numerous balancing poses that help improve steadiness with practice. I can really notice myself losing balance when I haven't practiced yoga in a few weeks; thankfully, it's a skill that comes back quickly.

Strive to incorporate stretching and balance-improving exercises when possible into the Week 10 workout schedule, below. Even a stretching session after a jog will help keep your muscles flexible—and will relax you.

Week 10 Workout Schedule

Monday	Tuesday	Wednesday	Thursday	Friday	Saturday	Sunday
1-hour walk or 30-minute jog	45 minutes strength	1-hour walk, 40-minute jog, or cardio class at gym	45 minutes strength	45-minute walk or jog, or cardio class at gym	Yoga or Pilates class	Rest

Awesome Balance Ball Workout for Total Body Strength

To do this workout, you will need an appropriately sized exercise ball. The ball makes the workout especially effective and works numerous muscles at once. Put on some fun music that will pump you up, and prop up your baby in a bouncy chair so she can watch you and be amazed with your strength. It is most effective if you warm up first for about five minutes by doing jumping jacks— or maybe by dancing around your house for a few minutes!

1. *Crunches.* Sit on the ball with your feet hip-width apart on the floor, keeping your back straight. With your core tightened, lean back until your abs are straining. Hold for three deep breaths, and then sit back up. Repeat 15 times.

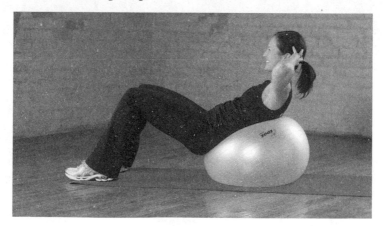

2. *Bridge.* Lie on the ground with your legs up on the ball from the knees down. Tighten your abs, and raise your hips and rear off the floor. Hold for three deep breaths. Be sure to contract your gluteal and hamstring muscles. Repeat 15 times.

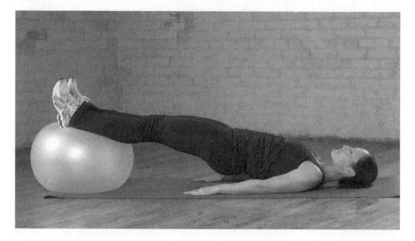

3. *Bridge with Hamstring Curl.* Stay in bridge position with your legs on the ball, lying on your back. Flex your buttocks and lift your hips off the floor, and then use your hamstrings to curl the ball slightly toward your rear while strengthening your core. Dig your heels into the ball and really engage your hamstring muscles. Hold for three seconds, and then relax and repeat the sequence ten times.

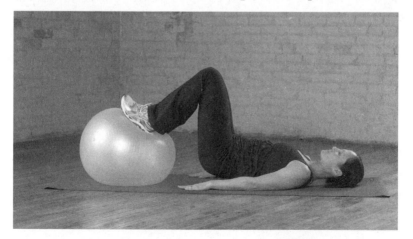

4. *Tick-Tocks.* Lie on the floor with the ball squeezed between your feet or shins. Use your abs to slowly lower your legs down to the left, keeping your shoulders on the floor. Bring your legs back to center and drop them to the right side. Be careful that your back does not arch. Repeat ten times on each side.

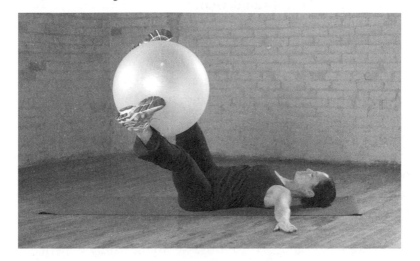

5. *Ball Plank Push-ups.* Start with your hands on the floor and your legs up on the ball on your lower shins. Do as many push-ups as you can, keeping your core tight. Do not arch your back!

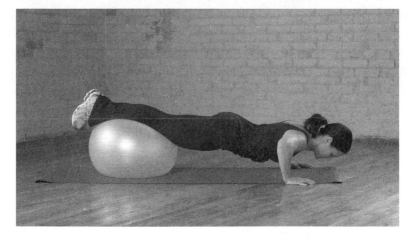

Sanity Saver: Balancing Doing with Being

Since becoming a mother, I have noticed that I have a tendency to move and "do" continually, both out of habit and necessity. Many of us are constantly moving, tidying, and doing things we feel must get done. It's understandable when running a household, working, raising children, and caring for a baby to feel like you have to be in motion 24 hours a day just to keep up. But you don't, and you shouldn't.

There is a time to do and a time to just "be." With a child now in grade school, I realize how short her time at home with me as a baby and toddler really was. I worked outside the home for much of it, which made it seem even more fleeting. You hear it all the time from older people: "Enjoy every minute with your kids because before you know it, they will be all grown up." I used to smile politely when I heard this and then go home to my chaotic house and piles of laundry. I would think, *I can't wait until my kids grow up and can do their own laundry and help around the house.* When we have thoughts like this, we are not fully experiencing and enjoying the little moments in our lives.

Concentrate on doing the tasks you must accomplish. For example, make a plan to spend an hour or so working on a project while your baby is napping or entertained. When the hour is up, you are done working; it is time to be with and enjoy your children or to relax and de-stress. You can multitask during the "doing" part of your life but not during the "being" part. When it is time to be, simply be completely present and experience your life. Fully immerse yourself in the little moments.

Affirmation for the Week

The quest for balance can be challenging for mothers; however, I will try to refresh myself every night while I sleep and start fresh in my pursuit of balance with each new day. What happened yesterday is in the past, and today is an opportunity to seek the life balance that brings me the most satisfaction and joy.

I have the power to create my life in a way that achieves balance, by managing my time to fit in the activities and people that mean the most to me. Living my life in alignment with my priorities will bring me the greatest sense of satisfaction, so I will do my best to spend my energy and time on the things that really matter to me. I will reorganize my life as needed to better serve my pursuit of balance and to experience more joy in my everyday life.

★☐★

Claim Your Mama Mojo

"Let your joy be unconfined!"

— MARK TWAIN

I remember the day I knew I had gotten my mojo back after having my first child. I was visiting my family and had left the baby at home to run some errands by myself. I had actually gone running that morning, returned home, showered, and gotten ready. Then I went out on my own after nursing the baby. I felt alive, alert, and free! I went into a coffee shop to grab a beverage. While I was there, a college-aged man came up and flirted with me. Once I realized what was happening, I am sure I got a silly grin on my face. I had felt fat and frumpy for so long that finding out someone who didn't know me considered me attractive gave me incredible happiness and hope. It sounds silly, I know, but I realized at that moment that I still "had it." You still have "it," too.

Of course, there were countless occasions after that moment when I felt as though I had lost my mojo again. There were even days when I felt as though I would never get it back. But I worked hard to restore my mojo because it was so important to me. I have seen countless women struggling to get their mojo back after having babies. It's natural to struggle after such a life- and body-changing event.

Mama mojo is that sexy self-confidence that only mothers can have. It's just a slightly different softness and strength that the people around you can sense. You have this beautiful mojo within, and if you don't feel it at this moment, don't worry. By the end of this week, you will be radiating your mojo in a way that is alluring to everyone around you.

Mamas who express their mojo are unstoppable. They have confidence, knowledge, and understanding that are gained from loving children so deeply. These women possess previously untapped potential that is somehow released during motherhood. Have you heard of marathon runners who become faster with each child or women who don't only do well after maternity leave but quickly leap to new heights? I personally don't think this new power is biochemical or physical; rather, it comes from deep inner strength.

What are the characteristics of a woman who has gotten her mojo back? She is joyful, smiles a lot, is friendly, walks with good posture, and exudes confidence. She has a love of life and a sense of adventure, laughs easily, and is simply fun to be around. Some people were born with huge quantities of mojo; others of us have to work at it. We all have the capability of regaining and exuding mojo, including you. Have you gotten your mama mojo going yet? It's time to let it flow!

Knowing You've Got It

A central component of mojo is self-confidence. We all know women who are confident and sassy, whether they have "perfect" bodies or not. They generally walk with great posture and exude poise and positive energy. Men find women who are confident very sexy, just as women find confident men sexy. When my husband comes home in his Air Force flight suit with his head held high, he radiates strength and confidence, and I find it completely sexy (as I am guessing women do everywhere he goes). Men who wear uniforms for work often do it with pride, which is why women have such a weakness for men in uniform.

A perfect example of women who exude confidence is belly dancers. I was recently mesmerized by a belly-dancing recital at a festival in my small town. The belly dancers were all very curvy and womanly, wearing midriff-baring outfits and bedazzled with jewels around their waists. Not one of them was model material, yet they were so beautiful. The way they moved their bodies was very sensual, and the very act of what they were doing seemed to make them comfortable in their own skin. Their body comfort and ease at shaking their hips in public were so inspiring.

You do still have it; you just have to *know* you have it. It's there within you, possibly buried by exhaustion, a few extra pounds, and a lack of practice. Getting enough rest and taking time to care for yourself are the first steps to getting your mojo back. Remember, you do not have to look or be perfect in any way to exude confidence!

Fake It Until You Make It!

You might not be feeling your most confident at the moment, but this is where I recommend the old adage, "Fake it until you make it." When you are not happy, for instance, if you smile and force yourself to think happy thoughts, you will actually begin to cheer up. The same thing happens with confidence. Take the time to put on a little makeup, dress in something you feel cute in, and walk with good posture and your head held high! Suddenly, you might actually find yourself feeling confident, as well.

Who cares if you are a bit over your ideal weight or have a little pudge on your belly? Who else even knows that you have stretch marks? And really, who cares, besides you? My husband didn't notice the stretch marks on the underside of my breasts for years, until I stupidly pointed them out. I was self-conscious about them, but he didn't even see them. When you truly love yourself, you radiate something that is attractive because we all (whether we are conscious of it or not) have a desire to love ourselves.

Have faith in yourself and your abilities, and be proud of all that you and your body have accomplished. Once you focus on your good traits, you will have an easier time carrying yourself with a confident grace that everyone around you will find captivating.

The Art of Flirting with Your Man

We can all use an ego boost from time to time. That's why you should put your sexy mojo into flirting with your husband. I know that women flirt with my husband; he's a tall, dark, handsome fighter pilot, so I can completely understand why. However, I want to be the one who flirts with him the most and the best. I am the one who knows his weaknesses and what he needs to hear, so I can boost his ego better than any other woman. I want him to get enough attention from me that he doesn't need any from other women to feel good about himself.

Flirting is a fun way to engage with your man and use the coquettish skills that you hope you still have. It's important to let him know that you are still crazy about him. Work to keep him interested in you, as though you have just started dating. It is essential that you "date" your husband throughout your marriage, to keep the spark alive. Our husbands see us so many times at our worst while we are pregnant and have newborns, so take the opportunity to look and feel your best. This gives you the confidence to talk to your man in a flirty, suggestive way—like you did back in the beginning.

What worked on him back then? Was it flirty e-mails, a perfume that drove him crazy, or a certain look that made him melt? Think back to the things you used to win him over, and do them now. Hone your flirting skills so that he is one happy husband, and your marriage will be strengthened.

One Hot Mama's Top Ten Flirting Techniques

1. Smile.
2. Make eye contact.
3. Pay attention and focus on what he says.
4. Be interesting.
5. Dress in a way you know he likes.
6. Listen.
7. Smell amazing.
8. Wear something sexy underneath, and let him know.
9. Compliment him authentically and generously.
10. Show sincere appreciation.

Put the O Back in "MOM"!

I wish I could take credit for this cute little phrase, but I found it on the website for Mama Gena's School of Womanly Arts (**www .mamagenas.com**). I have not graduated from this school, but it is certainly on my bucket list. Mama Gena's mission is to "enhance and expand the voice of women by fanning the flames of their desires, which opens the doors of fun and pleasure for everyone." Mama Gena and I both agree that women who are in touch with their desires can bring more passion to all areas of life.

Motherhood might equal frumpy and sexless to some. But in my mind, it equals confidence and sensuality in an entirely new, beautiful, maternal-goddess kind of way. Use the motherhood experience as a catalyst to give you the confidence to go after what you really want, both sexually and in the rest of your life. Your sex life could probably use a little boost after all the ups and downs of late pregnancy and the period right after childbirth. Now is the time to spice things back up and ask for what you really want in bed. Trust me, men find assertive women to be quite a turn-on.

This confident seductress in the bedroom will pleasantly surprise your partner.

It's important to understand what happens in your body during an orgasm. Your pubococcygeus (PC) muscle, the hammock-like muscle that supports your pelvic organs, contracts. You can locate this muscle by stopping the flow of urine, midstream. After giving birth, this can be tougher to do! This muscle can become weakened and damaged during the birth process, so it is crucial to strengthen it using Kegel exercises (described earlier in the book). If you want stronger orgasms, you need to have a stronger PC!

It's important to get into a sexy frame of mind if you want to achieve orgasm as often as possible. Getting enough sleep and getting yourself "in the mood" before joining your husband in bed can really help this process. You have been working hard on your body and on becoming more confident, so use this to your advantage in the bedroom. You are beautiful and attractive, and I promise that you can get your mama mojo back in the bedroom, too. You and your husband will both be much better off for it!

Arouse Your Adventurous Spirit

You will know you've got your mojo back when you have a desire for adventure. If you are not feeling this, plan to do something adventurous either by yourself or as a date with your partner. It will get your adrenaline pumping again and reignite your zest for life. What does adventure mean? It means doing something exciting and out of the ordinary. When you have a new baby, adventurous might mean going out for a drink and to an action flick in the middle of the day—while during your younger days, adventure meant going on a backpacking excursion in Central America. It's certainly relative, but the point is to do something that increases your pulse and makes you feel invigorated!

By nature, most men love excitement and challenge, so a life partner who is adventurous and loves life is not only ideal but super sexy. Motherhood can make you want to go into safe mode, but see if you can challenge yourself to embrace the adventurer within.

Here are a few ideas for adventurous dates with your partner:

- Go on a hike in the wild and make it extra exciting by making out or even doing something more intimate (use your imagination)

- Go rock climbing at an indoor climbing gym

- Check out a nearby town

- Try a new ethnic restaurant

- Go to a concert that you would not normally attend

- Go mountain biking, kayaking, sailing, downhill skiing, or snowboarding

- Visit a shooting range or batting cage

Start dreaming of the adventurous things you want to do one day on a bigger and grander scale. Being the mother of a new baby might not be the time for crazy adventures, but you can start dreaming of your next major trip that you will take when your children are old enough. Develop an adventure "bucket list" that makes your heart rate increase and gets you excited. Is it traveling to exotic countries and experiencing unknown cultures? Is it bungee jumping or scuba diving in clear, warm waters? It is sailing around the world? Dream big, and write down anything that comes to mind, no matter how far out it might seem. Here are a few crazy, wild, "someday" adventure ideas:

- Going on an African safari

- Climbing Mt. Kilimanjaro

- Visiting an ashram in India

- Sailing around the Caribbean on a chartered yacht

- Going to a week-long yoga, spa, or meditation retreat

- Cruising around the Galapagos Islands

- Heli-skiing

- Parasailing

- Hang gliding

- Driving a racecar

- Traveling across Europe with your best friend or husband

- A biking trip, vineyard tour, or culinary class in Italy or France

- Attending a surf school

- Touring and volunteering in a developing country

- Learning to scuba dive, and then planning an exotic diving vacation

- Learning to speak another language, and then planning a trip to use your skills

Revive Your Sense of Humor

Having a baby can bring out your serious side and make life seem heavy with responsibility. When you've got your mojo back, you will know it because you will be able to find humor in stressful and often gross situations. If you make light of some of the difficult times parenting can bring, life will become more fun for everyone.

I remember one day when my daughter had a serious diarrhea blowout all over her adorable outfit, her blankets, and the car seat. What a mess! There was poop everywhere, and I just wanted to cry. As I was trying to wash off my screaming baby in the tub while surrounded by poopy, smelly clothes, my husband walked in from work and said with a smile, "Shitty day, huh?" I burst out laughing. That was just what I needed; it really was a humorous situation. Imagining what I looked like was definitely funny. I even had poop on my cheek. As mothers, we will experience many difficult and sometimes super gross situations with babies . . . all you can do is laugh.

Having a sense of humor and laughing easily are very attractive qualities. In fact, telling a well-timed and witty joke will make your spouse think you are both funny and intelligent. Men also love it when women laugh at their jokes. What a fun place your house will be with more smiling and laughter. We all like people who can laugh at themselves when it's warranted. When you do something brainless because you are exhausted, make a joke of it. Why not? It's probably pretty darn funny. Your baby will also do things that are cute and funny; laugh easily, and it will teach your children to do the same. But never make fun at someone else's expense. You are smart enough to recognize the difference; you will know when people can be laughed with and when they're not up for it. Have fun!

Nourishment: Eating for Joy!

Dieting and trying to lose weight can take the joy out of eating. I believe that delicious food is one of life's delights, and it should be enjoyed with others! By delicious food, I don't mean fast food or fatty, fried food. I mean a meal cooked with love, savored with friends or family, and perhaps enjoyed with a fabulous glass of wine.

Preparing meals when you have a baby can take on a new sense of duty, which can start to feel like a drag. A long day at work, or at home with a needy baby, can make meal preparation seem like yet another task on your already long to-do list. See if you can convince your spouse to take on dinner one or two nights a week. Plan on getting takeout or eating out one or two nights, if you can afford it. Then you really have just three or four nights of meal planning to contend with. You might be more inclined to do it well if you don't feel pressure every night of the week.

I challenge you to actually enjoy everything you put in your mouth for a day. You might see this as a free ticket to make poor food choices, but I am challenging you to eat *healthfully* while loving every bite. It is entirely possible. Healthy foods can be prepared in ways that taste amazing, without adding a lot of fat. Foods with certain spices and combinations of ingredients are so delightful that you won't even recognize them as "health food." People who have adopted healthy eating enjoy their food (if prepared well) just as much as those who consume a fattening, high-calorie diet.

Getting inspired to try new food preparations can bring the fun back to cooking. Here are a few ways to prepare wonderfully tasty food without adding too much fat:

- Poaching, baking, broiling, or grilling fish

- Grilling or broiling meat

- Using exotic spices

- Using enough salt (if you don't have a blood pressure problem)

- Using healthier fats, such as olive oil, when sautéing vegetables

- Substituting applesauce for a portion of the oil when baking

- Adding just a little cheese

Fitness: Fun Workouts

Exercising can be incredibly fun. Do you believe me yet? Zumba, kick boxing, and spinning classes, or walking with a friend, can be truly enjoyable. This entire week is about experiencing more pleasure in your daily life, so extend this challenge to your workouts. Maybe the key is finding a lively aerobics instructor who somehow makes time fly. The best instructors have infectious energy and awesome music; you leave their classes invigorated.

Keep trying new workouts until you finish one with a satisfied smile on your face.

A big part of what makes exercise feel like such a chore for many women is boredom. Maybe you just need to do something completely new and exciting. Or maybe you are exerting yourself so hard at the gym that you are miserable the entire time. There is definitely a place for pushing yourself if you are trying to improve your fitness level, but there also needs to be a place for enjoyable workouts.

If you are drawing a blank, think of the activities you enjoyed as a child. Did you love to swim or dance? What's stopping you from doing these things now? Maybe running miles on end has become a form of drudgery for you, which indicates to me that you need to mix in other exercises a few days a week. I have heard women say they don't do Zumba or other dance-based workouts because they don't seem like a good enough workout. The truth is that a 140-pound woman will burn approximately 500 calories per hour during a moderate-level Zumba class (**www.zumbacalories .com**), which is the equivalent of running about five miles. That's not too shabby! I am not saying you should do only these fun, dancing types of workouts; just mix it up so you don't get bored.

Other fun workouts include:

- Hula hooping
- Belly dancing
- Trampoline workouts
- Hip-hop dancing
- Ballroom dancing
- Pole dancing
- Martial arts
- Ballet
- Hiking or biking with someone fun

- In-line skating, roller-skating, and ice-skating
- Rock climbing
- Beach volleyball
- Team softball
- Wii Fit
- Racquetball
- Skiing, snowboarding, and snowshoeing
- Old-fashioned aerobics classes with good music

Try to incorporate a few of the fun ideas presented in this section into your workouts this week. Remember all of the benefits of working out, such as looking and feeling your sexiest, and let those thoughts push you just a little harder. Also make sure to have at least a few enjoyable workouts each week, so they become something you look forward to and want to make a priority in your busy schedule.

Week 11 Workout Schedule

Monday	Tuesday	Wednesday	Thursday	Friday	Saturday	Sunday
1-hour walk or 45-minute jog	45 minutes strength	1-hour walk, 45-minute jog, or cardio class at gym	45 minutes strength	45-minute walk or jog, or cardio class at gym	Yoga or Pilates class	Rest

Get Your Mojo Moving Workout

First of all, crank up the music. If you haven't already, create a fantastic playlist that you can hardly sit still to. Dance around the house for at least ten minutes for your warm-up.

1. *Hip Circles.* This move is self-explanatory! Make it fun, and really loosen up your hips and lower back. Roll your neck at the same time if it feels good.

2. *Squat Swing.* Start by standing with your feet a bit wider than shoulder-width apart, holding a single dumbbell with both hands out in front of your hips. Squat down until your knees are parallel to the floor as you swing the dumbbell down between your legs. Quickly stand up, swinging the dumbbell forward and then up over your head as you lift your left leg straight from out to the side, keeping your toes pointed forward. Lower your left foot to floor and return to the deep squat, bringing the dumbbell back between your legs. Repeat the sequence with your right leg, doing 10 to 15 repetitions on each leg.

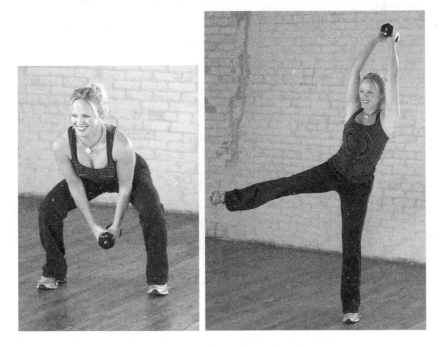

3. *Bound Angle Pose.* Start by sitting with your legs out in front of you, and then pull your heels in toward your pelvis while

dropping your knees to the side. Bring the soles of your feet to-gether and press your legs gently toward the floor. Hold the posi-tion for at least one minute.

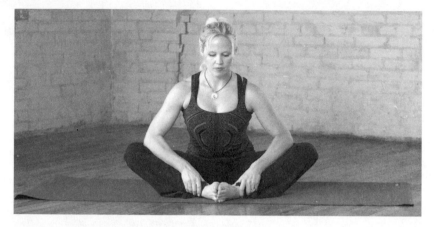

4. *Plow Pose.* Start by lying on your back. Using your abdomi-nal muscles, lift your legs up over your head and keep extending until your toes touch the floor behind your head. Lace your fingers and keep your arms straight, pressing into the floor. Be sure that your hips are aligned over your shoulders. Hold the pose for five exhalations or as long as you can. As you come out of the pose, roll out one vertebra at a time with your legs straight.

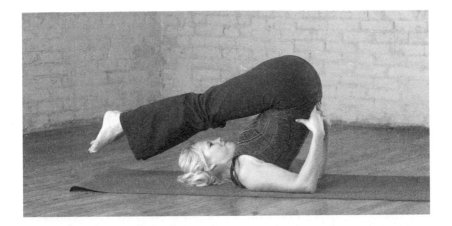

5. *Camel Pose*. Begin this pose by kneeling on the floor with your knees hip-width apart. Rest your hands on the back of your pelvis, bases of the palms on the tops of the buttocks, fingers pointing down. Reach your hands back one at a time to grasp your heels and bring your hips forward so that they are over your knees. Let your head fall back, opening your throat. Hold this pose for five breaths or up to a minute.

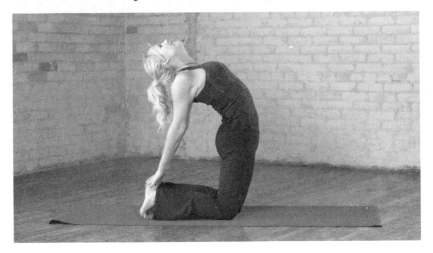

Sanity Saver: A Sexy Night Out

I know I have talked a lot about going on dates with your partner and rekindling the flame in your marriage, but this is a little different. This sanity saver takes things to a whole new level. Now that you've got your mojo back, you can plan a different kind of date . . . one with a little more flirtation and spice. I am presenting this as a sanity saver because if you do this type of sexy, fun dating with your husband, you will most likely avoid serious marital problems (unless you are married to a real jerk, which I doubt you are). By going on these kinds of dates, both of you will more feel secure and fulfilled in your marriage and more self-confident overall.

Take as long as you need to get ready for your date. Start during naptime if you have to, and be sure to shave, pluck, and do things to make yourself look and feel sexy, as time allows. I have three children, so I know how difficult this can be, but do your best. If you need to, have your babysitter come a little early so you can get ready in peace. Put on the sexiest undergarments you own. Even better, wear a garter under a skirt with a thong. Do these things as much for yourself as for your man. Make sure you smell really, really good. Wear that perfume that your husband comments on every time. Get yourself in the mind-set of a confident man-eater.

Start the date at a bar or somewhere you and your husband would have gone when you were dating—and no kidding, flirt with your man. Not just the innocent, friendly, unintentional type of flirting; I am talking about the "I want you and want to have your babies" kind. You clearly have the skills; you have a baby, don't you? You may just need to remind yourself.

Here are a few tips for this mojo revival date:

- Make sure he can see cleavage or leg, whichever asset you feel most confident about.

- Sit close enough so he can smell you.

- Lean in toward him.

- Make eye contact.

- Focus completely on him.

- Listen to what he says intently.

- Laugh at his jokes.

- Earlier in the day, read the paper, watch a little network news, check out *The New York Times* online, or listen to NPR, so you have an idea about what's going on in the world and have a few non-baby topics to discuss.

- Order an absolutely delicious dinner, but don't eat so much that you will have indigestion or any stomach issues afterward . . . which can make bedroom time less enjoyable.

- Touch him a lot.

- Kiss his neck in the car.

- Make out in the car.

- See if other things can happen . . . in the car.

- If not, make your way inside, tell your babysitter good night, and then head straight to bed.

- Keep yourself in the mind-set of wanting your man and nothing else, because tonight you are a sex goddess.

Affirmation for the Week

My sensuality as a woman did not die the moment I gave birth; in fact, I can feel more empowered now that I have accomplished such a feat. I have the potential to be sexier than ever, although it might take a little additional effort now that my time and energy are pulled in more directions. I consider my sex life to be a crucial part my romantic relationship. I will not let it go by the wayside.

The first step in reclaiming my mojo is to take exceedingly good care of myself. I understand that sometimes it will be difficult to feel sexy when I am so exhausted and drained that I can't imagine "doing the deed." However, I will do my best to take care of my body, mind, and soul in a way that helps me have a positive body image. And I will try to preserve energy for maintaining my love life and for living my best life overall.

★☐★

You Are Fabulous!

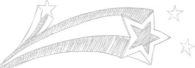

*"The purpose of life is to live it, to taste experience to
the utmost, to reach out eagerly and without fear
for newer and richer experience."*

—ELEANOR ROOSEVELT

I had the honor recently of hearing an amazing woman speak
about her near-death experience, including her unspoken conversations with God while on her deathbed. The woman's name is
Anita Moorjani. She was dying from stage IV cancer, her body rid-
den with dozens of tumors. As she lay in the hospital in a coma,
her body swollen and systematically shutting down from organ
failure, she was given the choice to join God and let go of her
suffering or to rejoin her husband and live. There is so much to
the story, but the thing that God told her to let all people know
was that they are beautiful and perfect just the way they are. During Anita's near-death experience, she received an innate knowing
that God loves us all so much and just wants us to love ourselves
and live in a way that honors the amazing gift of life.

When I talked to Anita up close, I felt a strong force of love
and kindness radiating from her. She embodied pure love, and
despite not being an extrovert, she has chosen to speak publicly to
try to spread the messages she heard from God—specifically, that
we were all born to be magnificent and that life is a precious gift.
Anita's new book, detailing her grave illness, her near-death journey, and her complete recovery, is called *Dying to Be Me*.

We can all live as though each moment is a treasure. It may not feel like it when we are folding laundry, scrubbing the floor, or dealing with a child's tantrum, but these are all uniquely human experiences. So are inhaling the sweet scent of your baby's hair, feeling the body heat of a precious sleeping child, hugging someone you love, laughing with a friend, and enjoying a delicious meal. We can choose how we experience each moment, and sometimes we just have to remind ourselves that it's all a gift: the bad and the good.

You *are* absolutely fabulous, and when you find yourself criticizing your body, your looks, or the way you are, you are dishonoring yourself and everything you've been blessed with. If you don't like something about yourself, the best thing you can do is love yourself enough to try to make it better.

You Are Beautiful

You might not always feel it, but you are completely beautiful. Physical beauty is one thing, and beauty that radiates from within is another. Have you met someone who was what society might label "average," but she dressed well, took great care of herself, and gave off such loveliness and strength that she became prettier to you each time you came into contact with her? That's the true beauty that lasts a lifetime.

Motherhood can make feeling beautiful more of a challenge. There are times when I look in the mirror after a hectic day home with my kids or after a sleepless night with sick children and criticize the bags under my eyes or the appearance of a new wrinkle. It can be tough to look in the mirror and think, *Wow, I am pretty!* Take a little additional time for yourself on those days, applying a little extra concealer and brighter lipstick, until you are satisfied with what you see in the mirror.

Beauty is a loaded word, and knowing you are a beautiful woman despite the extra pounds, new wrinkles, and perceived imperfections is an expression of self-love. Stop the self-criticism, and do what you need to do to feel pretty. Smiling is one of the first things you can do to make yourself more beautiful. Research supports this; in fact, a smile is one of the top things that triggers attraction in the human brain's medial orbitofrontal cortex, which is the reward center of the brain.[1]

Do you need easy ideas on how you can feel more beautiful? Here are a few suggestions to help make your outside as beautiful as your inside:

- Smile.

- Wear lipstick or gloss.

- Wear earrings.

- Take the time to apply lotion to your entire body after a bath.

- Wear perfume or body oil, even when you're just staying home all day.

- Paint your nails; or even better, get a manicure and pedicure.

- Get a haircut, highlights, or blowout. You will feel prettier immediately.

- Have your makeup applied professionally at a department store.

- Use good facial products. Effective cleansers, eye creams, and night creams can help your skin look refreshed and well-rested, even when you're not. Drug stores sell cheaper products that have the same active ingredients as their more expensive department store counterparts!

- Get rid of clothes you don't like, and make room in your closet to slowly purchase clothes that fit and flatter (especially after losing your baby weight).

- If it fits your budget, visit a personal shopper at a nice department store. It's free, and the stylist can help you pick out clothes that flatter you and that you might not have chosen for yourself.

- Get a sassy, sexy new pair of shoes. You don't have to spend a lot of money. There are great, fashionable shoes at Payless!

You Are Creative

You have so much creative potential simmering within you. We all have innate imaginative brilliance in some form, but we are raised to depend on our more logical left brain to the point that we lose touch with our more creative right brain. Each of us is born with a tendency to be left- or right-brained. It is believed that the left hemisphere of the brain is in charge of our abilities to be analytical and objective, while the right hemisphere is responsible for our abilities to be creative, intuitive, and feeling. Have you ever known a child who hates to paint or draw? While we might be born with a tendency to be more right- or left-brained, I believe that we all have the ability to learn to be more balanced with regard to use of the hemispheres of the brain. Society often focuses on nurturing the left brain through math, science, and being analytical. These skills are valued because they tend to help you make more money as an adult; however, it is usually more enjoyable to live with greater balance between the left and right brain hemispheres.

As a child, I was considered creative. I loved to write stories and use my imagination. As I grew up, I focused on becoming an engineer and a scientist, because I believed I could be more "successful" in life by utilizing the related skills. Although applying math skills was not nearly as fun to me as being creative, I was able to train myself to become left-brain dominant. I actually started to believe that I was not creative at all. I did not attempt any creative projects in my 20s because I was so career focused. I convinced myself that I was analytical, and I believed it for many years. I have witnessed the same thing happen to some of my girlfriends, as well. Many of us have worked in male-dominated fields, where women are more respected when they operate as left-brainers.

Motherhood made me want to reclaim my right brain. I have seen this occur for many women. All of a sudden, we feel the spark of creativity that has been stifled—and we realize we might actually have a little more time at home to hone our creative skills. I used to think that my right-brained, creative friends were just the ones who were artists or fantastic decorators. I sold myself short. One day I realized that I have been a writer my entire life—and I had discounted writing as a creative endeavor. Once I started writing again, other creative ideas and abilities began to appear.

Do you consider yourself right-brain dominant or left-brain dominant? Is this true? If you have been staying home doing nothing but crafts and kid things, is there a part of you craving some intellectual stimulation? If you have been working in a high-powered, male-dominated, analytical type of career, is there some part of you that wants to be more expressive? Just consider balance. We often let ourselves get taken through life without a lot of our input until we become aware one day that we are completely out of alignment with who we truly are.

Here are a few ideas to help you reignite your creative spirit:

— *Start writing in a journal.* I have written in a journal on and off since the first grade, and no other act has helped me understand myself more. Sometimes when I am upset with my husband, I write in my journal to sort through my thoughts. I often realize that I am not actually mad about the matter at hand. Rather, I discover that I have been harboring anger about an unresolved conflict that occurred days prior, and something small triggered my resentment. Without journaling, I might not have understood these feelings and figured myself out.

— *Get some special paper and paints, and see what happens.* Being left-brained for so long, when I tried this, I had to follow the steps in a book on how to watercolor. The final product was actually pretty, and it empowered me to try something on my own. I have learned that I have little painting skill, but it was really fun!

— *Do a craft.* I have never considered myself crafty, and I grew up to believe that it wasn't my "thing" because I was a career woman. While I can't claim to have a lot of talent in this area, I really enjoy doing little projects on my own and with my children when I have extra time.

— *Cook creatively.* Get out of your comfort zone in the kitchen, and try something new. Challenge yourself by trying a recipe out of *Gourmet* magazine or an ethnic recipe.

— *Peruse creative blogs or Pinterest for inspiration.* I may not always have creative ideas myself, but I have learned that all of my most creative friends seek inspiration from others for many of their projects. There is nothing wrong with getting ideas from others! There are amazing and talented people out there who blog about their projects related to sewing, decorating, writing, cooking, gift wrapping, inspiration, etc.

— *Get a new magazine.* The next time you walk through the grocery store checkout, pick up a Martha Stewart magazine or something else that attracts you. Even better, large bookstores like Barnes and Noble have amazing magazine sections where you can find a publication on virtually any topic or hobby.

— *Take a class.* Take a painting, writing, or dance class! Stretch and challenge yourself to do something new and fun. While we were living in Florida, our Air Force squadron did monthly get-togethers (aka "coffees"), where we did fun and creative things like painting pottery (while sipping drinks). Gather a group of girl-friends and try something together. You might even take a sewing or acting class. Dang, I am inspiring myself to try something crazy and new! Knitting classes, anybody?

— *Start a blog.* If you enjoy writing or photography, blogging can be an incredible outlet. There are numerous free or inexpensive templates that make it very easy. You could consider blogging a challenge to sharpen your skills and share yourself with the world! I really enjoy cooking and craft blogs featuring beautiful photographs. While it may seem as though there is already a blog for everything, there is no blog with your unique viewpoint and spin on the world. Maybe there should be.

You Are Intelligent

Being pregnant and giving birth can do a little temporary brain damage (yes, it is temporary!), which I believe is largely related to exhaustion and hormone fluctuations. You are still smart, and in fact, some believe that the process of giving birth and raising babies improves women's brains. Katherine Ellison, author of *The Mommy Brain: How Motherhood Makes Us Smarter*, presents compelling evidence that, in many respects, motherhood does make us more capable and intelligent in the areas of perception, efficiency, resilience, motivation, and emotional intelligence. Ellison presents persuasive proof, supported by both human and animal studies, on how mothers outperform non-mothers in each of these categories. Perhaps you've lost a little confidence in your intellectual competency, but if you are reading this book, I know you have brilliance within.

If anything, the fire of your intellect might just need to be stoked a bit. There are countless ways to do this, but reading and learning something new are two of the best and most effective methods. Look for a book that will challenge your brain, such as historical fiction, the biography of someone you have always admired, or a thriller. Ask around about books that are thrilling and will keep you awake! Any new mom knows that a book has to keep her attention or else she will fall right asleep.

Learn something, such as a foreign language or a new technology. When I had my first child, I started losing confidence in my abilities as a scientist. I began reading technical journals again, and it really reengaged me. I was also intrigued and excited by my new iPhone and computer, and I took it as a challenge to learn everything I could about them. Research new and fun smartphone applications. If you are still working, learn about something technical that is completely out of your area of expertise. Challenge yourself!

You Are Loved

The mere fact that you are alive indicates that you are important. You may not always feel loved, but there are people out there who love you deeply. Believe this: I love you! The universe loves you! Your baby loves you! Knowing you are loved can make your entire experience of life more enjoyable—and can allow you to give love more freely yourself.

What Do You Believe About Yourself?

I am: two simple words with so much power. "I am" is one of the few things God calls himself in the Torah and the Bible. The great Indian sage Sri Ramana Maharshi also said, "'I am' is the name of God . . . God is none other than the Self."

How would you describe yourself, physically and otherwise? How do you usually follow the words, "I am"? The language you use to describe yourself is incredibly influential on your reality. You might have "I am" statements that you make out loud, as well as ones you say only to yourself. Your subconscious mind does not differentiate between reality and the chatter in your head; it believes whatever it hears.

I heard my five-year-old say, "I'm stupid" this morning, and it made me so sad. She is a perfectionist, and when she can't do things just right, she lashes out at herself. Most of us do. I find myself saying terrible things in my mind from time to time, such as, "I am such a moron" (when I forget something). If you tell yourself, "I am so forgetful," your brain will follow suit and behave forgetfully. If you have convinced yourself that you are fat, you will probably sabotage your efforts to lose weight.

Based on a few very valid situations where I lost valuable items, I was convinced and was repeatedly told that I lost things as a child. Therefore, I believed that I lost things for most of my life—and so I did. One day I purchased some expensive sunglasses, and I repeated to myself, "I don't lose things." Sure enough, I've had the sunglasses for nearly three years and really haven't lost anything since. Our thoughts are so powerful!

The words *I am* are powerful in so many ways. Make sure you use them with care and love. Start living with the end in mind, saying the things you are and those you wish to be, such as:

I am kind.

I am creative.

I am intelligent.

I am beautiful.

I am fit.

I am healthy.

I am powerful.

I am fun.

I am generous.

I am a good mother.

I am a great wife.

I am loved.

And you are!

A Little on the Law of Attraction

As you complete this book and go on with your fabulous life, I want to leave you with an understanding of the law of attraction. Boiled down, the law of attraction is the belief that like attracts like—meaning that the things you put positive energy toward will result in positive outcomes, and the things you put negative energy toward will result in negative results. For example, if you want to be wealthy but in your head and out loud you are always saying how broke and poor you are, you will most likely remain broke and poor. Likewise, if you'd like to be thin but every time you look at yourself in the mirror you think about how fat and disgusting your body is, you will have a difficult time ever reaching your ideal weight. Overcoming habitual thought patterns is very difficult, which is why most of us never reach our ideal weight or the point where we have enough money to feel completely comfortable.

I am not here to discuss whether the law of attraction is a real law based on quantum physics, but I can say with confidence and through experience that any human who changes his or her thought patterns from negative to positive will realize positive outcomes. Repeatedly visualizing a goal as if you have already attained it conditions your mind to believe it is possible. Over time, as that conditioning takes root through repetition, your belief leads you to act differently on many levels.

The law of attraction has been known for centuries and used by many of the world's great sages and leaders. It became more formalized in the early 1900s by what was called the New Thought Movement, popularized by William Walker Atkinson's 1906 book *Thought Vibration or the Law of Attraction in the Thought World* (available online at **http://gitacademy.tripod.com/GodsIn Training/ThoughtVibration.htm**).

Read the following quotes to understand that the idea of the law of attraction has been around for centuries and is not just a New Age belief:

"Therefore I tell you, whatever you ask for in prayer, believe that you have received it, and it will be yours."
—The Bible, Mark 11:24, approximately 70 A.D.

"Ask and it will be given to you; seek and you will find; knock and the door will be opened to you."
—The Bible, Matthew 7:7, approximately 70 A.D.

"Experiences are preceded by mind, led by mind, and produced by mind. If one speaks or acts with an impure mind, suffering follows even as the cartwheel follows the hoof of the ox . . .

If one speaks or acts with a pure mind, happiness follows like a shadow that never departs."
—Buddha, The Dhammapada, 1:1–2, 5th century A.D.

"When we come to see that Thought is a force—a manifestation of energy—having a magnet-like power of attraction, we will begin to understand the why and wherefore of many things that have heretofore seemed dark to us. There is no study that will so well repay the student for his time and trouble as the study of the workings of this mighty law of the world of Thought—the Law of Attraction."
—William Walker Atkinson, 1906

The law of attraction was popularized by the movie and book *The Secret*, which discussed the concept in three steps: ask, believe, and receive. I enjoyed the book and movie, but to me they over-simplified the process and focused too much on bringing material objects into your life while not focusing enough on the action required to accomplish this.

In my opinion, the law of attraction includes the following steps:

1. Become clear

2. Ask, and set your intention

3. Believe

4. Feel

5. Act

6. Let go

7. Receive

To help you understand these seven steps better, I will go into a little more detail about each of them and provide examples:

1. Become clear on what you really want. You might think that great wealth will solve all of your problems; however, I challenge you to really think about this and determine what would truly make your life better. Is it a healthier body? A larger home? A new car? I am not here to judge. If more money would make your life better, I want you to figure out exactly how much money it would take.

2. Ask the universe, God, Allah, Jesus, or whatever higher power(s) you believe in to bring into your life the situation or thing that you desire. **Set your intention** on obtaining this ideal every morning.

3. Believe that you can have whatever it is that you have asked for, and release all doubt and fear. This is one of the most critical steps. Let's say you really want to be debt free, but there is a little voice inside that doubts it is really possible. You might have a great deal of negative emotion associated with money because of the way you were raised, and it is difficult to overcome your fears. As long as doubt and fear exist in your heart, the desired outcome will probably not make its way into your life. The same applies when trying to get your body to its ideal weight. If you have a little negative voice within telling you that you will never be thin, then you probably won't be. Getting rid of fear and disbelief is difficult but very possible, with practice, prayer, and meditation. Retrain your brain to believe all things are possible!

4. Feel the way you'd feel if you had what you desire right now. Really imagine how you'd feel if you were debt free, if you lived in a nicer neighborhood, if you could pull on a size 6 dress with ease, or if you could be comfortable wearing a bikini at the beach. From all I have read and experienced, you need to live from the end in order to realize what you really want.

5. Acting is another crucial step in the process. You must take physical steps toward achieving your goal. Generally, you can't just put it out there that you want something and then have it granted without some sweat equity on your part. The magic happens when you do all of the steps—asking for the thing you want but making it clear that you aren't just wishing for it. Move in the direction of your ideal life, even if it's just baby steps, while believing fully that you will achieve it—and you will.

6. Let go to receive the full blessings that are lined up for you. This can be extremely difficult when you want something so badly! Have faith that, if you have made your wishes known and are working hard, everything you hope for will come your way in due time. If it doesn't, there is a very good reason. You have to believe that if you are meant to have something and are doing everything you can to make it happen, it will happen. Work hard, and watch amazing things start to materialize . . .

7. Receive the blessings and gifts that are meant for you. Accept them with such joy and gratitude that the universe can't help but give you more!

Nourishment: Sustainable Weight Loss

Maintaining a healthy, ideal weight is part of a lifestyle. Nobody can live on a diet, but you can make eating well and exercising an everyday part of your life. What will it take for you to sustain your weight loss and maintain your ideal weight?

There are a few people who do not need to exercise to maintain their ideal weight, but most of us will after a certain age. Exercising is important for many health reasons, and it will help your body have a more toned look, as well. As we have learned, getting enough sleep is also a crucial, if often overlooked, component of maintaining your ideal weight.

Recall the four key pieces to feeling fantastic, losing weight, and finally maintaining your ideal weight:

Adequate Sleep + Healthy Eating + Exercise + Body Love

These four things need to be part of your daily life—not just when you are trying to lose weight. I can guarantee that if you make sure you are practicing each of these four things, you will achieve and be able to maintain your weight loss.

Fitness: Making Exercise a Regular Part of Your Life

How do you feel about working out these days? Has it become part of your routine? Do you miss your workouts on days when you can't fit them in? Have you started enjoying exercising, or at least the way you feel afterward? Exercising is one of those things that will only get easier and more enjoyable with time. As you become more and more fit, you can branch out and try different types of workouts.

Here are a few memorable pieces of evidence to help you understand just how critical exercising is for your health and for avoiding being overweight.

- Medical professionals recommend 30 minutes per day of moderate exercise to prevent heart disease, but to lose weight or maintain weight loss, obesity experts say that you must exercise at least one hour most days of the week.

- In a study of the weight loss and maintenance histories of 34,000 women conducted by Harvard University, results showed that women who reported exercising an hour per day, five to six days per week, gained no or little weight over the 13-year study period.[2]

Exercising simply has to become part of your daily life in order for you to get the body you desire, to feel fabulous, and to remain as healthy as possible. Do what you have to so that you enjoy your daily workouts. If you despise running, try walking or gym classes. Keep experimenting with a variety of exercises until you find one that you enjoy and that makes you want to continue doing it. It will be one of the best things you can do in your life—for your confidence, energy level, and overall life satisfaction!

Ideally, the workout schedule for Week 12, below, is one you can strive to sustain indefinitely. Of course, there will be weeks when you just can't fit in all of the workouts, but use this schedule as a guideline to set your exercising goals. You might even find that you enjoy working out so much that you want to add time or workouts! If you train for a race or other event, you might need to work out even harder to prepare. Half marathon? Mountain climbing? You are now likely at a fitness level where you could start training for any of these types of challenging activities.

Week 12 Workout Schedule

Monday	Tuesday	Wednesday	Thursday	Friday	Saturday	Sunday
1-hour walk or 45-minute jog	45 minutes strength	1-hour walk or jog, or cardio class at gym	45 minutes strength	1-hour walk or jog, or cardio class at gym	Yoga or Pilates class	Rest

Everyday Quick Total Body Strengthener

This workout can be done on any of your strength days and will quickly work most major muscles. It is speedy and very effective! As always, warm up with a little jogging in place or dancing around the house. Go through this series of exercises three times.

1. *Lunge in Place with Bicep Curls.* Step forward into a lunge with your right leg forward and a five- to eight-pound weight in each hand. As you lower down until your thigh is parallel to the ground, simultaneously lift both weights from your sides up into a curl. Lower the weights back down as you straighten your legs. Do ten repetitions on each leg.

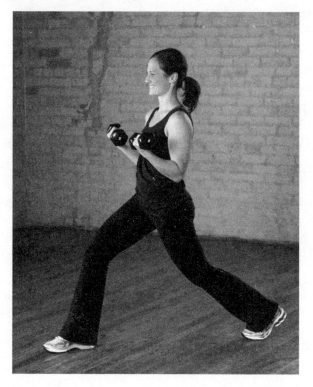

2. *Wide Stance Deadlift.* Stand with your feet hip-width apart and knees slightly bent. Hold a five- to eight-pound dumbbell in each hand, keeping your palms facing your body. Bend forward slowly while lowering the dumbbells to your upper shin. Use your gluteal muscles to slowly straighten to a standing position. Repeat 10 to 15 times.

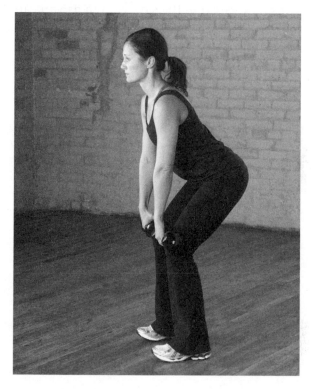

3. *Sumo Squat with Side Crunch and Knee Lift.* Start with your legs wider than hip width, holding a five- to eight-pound dumbbell or a medicine ball. Squat down until your thighs are as close to parallel to the floor as possible, holding the weight or ball straight down with both hands. Next, lift the weight or ball to your right shoulder while simultaneously crunching your right oblique and lifting your right knee up to the side as high as you can. Do 10 to 15 repetitions on the right and then switch sides.

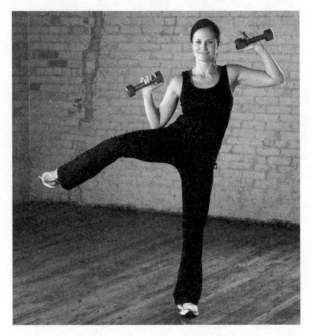

4. *Plié Squat with Overhead Triceps Curl.* Start with your legs in a plié position as shown, hands both clasping a five- to ten-pound dumbbell over your head. Lower your knees outward, but not over your toes, while lowering the weight behind your neck. Using your buttock and leg muscles, slowly straighten your legs while also lifting and straightening your arms. Repeat 10 to 15 times.

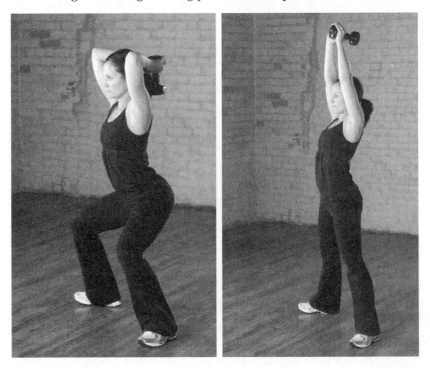

5. *Plank Hold with Front Arm Raises.* Start in a plank position with your arms directly below your shoulders. Keeping your neck neutral, tighten your core and raise your right arm straight in front of you to shoulder height and hold for a second before returning it to the ground. For an extra challenge, hold a light dumbbell in each hand. Repeat 10 to 15 times on each side.

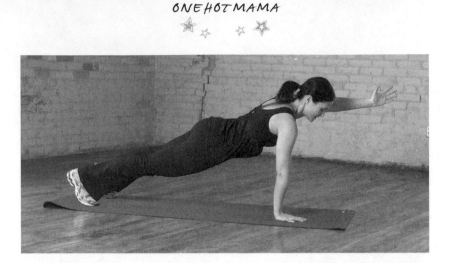

Be sure to follow the workout with a cool-down that includes some light stretching.

Sanity Saver: Surrounding Yourself with Positive Influences

As you continue on your motherhood journey, you need all the love, support, and positive energy possible. Of course, you can get positive energy from spiritual gurus, books, and blogs, but you also need real people in your life who encourage and uplift you. If you have a hard time thinking of friends who inspire you and make your life more joyful, it's time to use some of the ideas in this book to find a few new friends.

Have you met anyone recently who energized you, who really made you enjoy being in her presence? This is a soul friend—a soul sister. A person who brings out the best in you and inspires you to do bigger and better things is someone to value in your life and to spend as much time with as possible. A friend like this will lift you up when you're down, encourage you to take good care of yourself, and spark new ideas for how you can make your life better.

Does anyone in your family exert a negative influence on your life? If so, minimize your exposure to him or her. It can be difficult to choose to put distance between yourself and someone in your own family, but sometimes it is the healthiest thing you can do. You don't need to make a big deal out of it; rather, just quietly go on with your life with joy and freedom, sending the difficult family member love and forgiveness.

Do you have any friends right now who are catty, who spend their time talking poorly about others and gossiping? How does it make you feel to hear that? Do you ever find yourself participating? I have, and I have felt pretty disgusted with myself afterward. There are many people out there who are unaware of their dysfunction and the negative energy they release. These are not people who will help push you to be a better person or to live a better life. In fact, some of these friends might even be dragging you down.

You are amazing, and you deserve friends who bring out the best in you. You know who these people are. Cultivate supportive and positive relationships. These are the friends who will keep you sane and make your life much more fun.

Affirmation for the Week

I have so much going for me. I know that I am an intelligent, fun, beautiful, and special woman. I am also a wonderful mother! Like most women, I sometimes struggle with self-doubt, feeling overwhelmed, and being hard on myself. The key is to be aware of when my thoughts are negative and then turn them around. I will try to remember to be more aware of how I think and speak about myself. I know that I will become what I think about, and I need to be very mindful of how I follow the words, "I am." I am confident and creative, and I look forward to living each day of my balanced and joyful life.

★ ◻ ★

Month 3 Workout Schedule

	Monday	Tuesday	Wednesday	Thursday	Friday	Saturday	Sunday
Week 9	45-minute walk or 30-minute jog	30 minutes strength	1-hour walk, 40-minute jog, or cardio class at gym	30 minutes strength	45-minute walk, 30-minute jog, or cardio class at gym	Yoga or Pilates class	Rest
Week 10	1-hour walk or 30-minute jog	45 minutes strength	1-hour walk, 40-minute jog, or cardio class at gym	45 minutes strength	45-minute walk or jog, or cardio class at gym	Yoga or Pilates class	Rest
Week 11	1-hour walk or 45-minute jog	45 minutes strength	1-hour walk, 45-minute jog, or cardio class at gym	45 minutes strength	45-minute walk or jog, or cardio class at gym	Yoga or Pilates class	Rest
Week 12	1-hour walk or 45-minute jog	45 minutes strength	1-hour walk or jog, or cardio class at gym	45 minutes strength	1-hour walk or jog, or cardio class at gym	Yoga or Pilates class	Rest

AFTERWORD

It is my most sincere wish that this book has taken you through a life-transforming process and has helped you get back your best self, in both mind and body. I have said it many times throughout this book: Motherhood is a challenging experience that can keep you stressed, overwhelmed, and disheveled, or it can push you to greater heights. You can let raising children consume you and lose yourself in the process—or you can set an excellent example by living your very best life and taking good care of yourself, so that you have more love and energy for your partner and kids.

Since I finished writing this book, I have given birth to my third child and gone through the process of getting my mind and body back once again using the tried and true methods outlined in this book. I weighed in at four weeks postpartum, and to my dismay, I was 30 pounds over my ideal weight. Talk about a challenge to practice what I preach related to self-love! I know how hard it is to love a body that looks foreign and unsightly, and I know the overwhelming feeling of having a substantial amount of weight to lose. I have experienced feeling fat and have literally taken every measure described in this book to get re-centered, focused, happy, fit, and skinny once again! It's not easy, but it is entirely possible. I hope you have had a wonderful experience through this process, and I hope you will share it with me.

I encourage you to take a few minutes now to reflect on your experience over the past three months or however long your journey has been. Do you feel happier overall? Have you met your goals? Have you achieved your desired weight? Look back at what you wrote in the Introduction, and honor your successes. Celebrate your accomplishments, whether they are related to losing baby weight, setting and achieving goals, or simply becoming more joyful or centered in your daily living. Any part of your life that has improved as a result of reading this book is a success to me!

If you aren't at your ideal weight yet, simply continue to implement the techniques, eating habits, and workout schedules presented in the book. It can take time to get your body to where you want it, and slow and steady weight loss is the most healthy and sustainable kind. Hang in there, and stick with it!

I am grateful and honored to have been part of your journey, and I send you much love and light as you go on with your life as a mother. Please contact me at **erin@erincox.com** if you have any questions about the book or if there is anything else that I can do to support you.

I wasn't able to include absolutely everything I would have liked to in this book, which is why I have created a multitude of free resources on my website, **www.erincox.com**. You will find numerous useful and motivational materials, such as recipes, exercises, and online workshops. As a reader of this book, please use the code HOTMAMA to receive a 25 percent discount on the online course or coaching package of your choice.

★☆★

NOTES

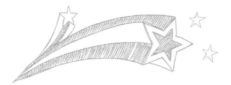

Week One

1. P. O. Anderson, "Alcohol and Breastfeeding," *Journal of Human Lactation* 11, no. 4 (1995): 321–323.

2. J. A. Mennella and G. K. Beauchamp, "The Transfer of Alcohol to Human Milk: Effects on Flavor and the Infant's Behavior," *New England Journal of Medicine* 325 (1991): 981–985.

3. L. Lamberg, "Rx for Obesity: Eat Less, Exercise More, and—Maybe—Get More Sleep," *The Journal of the American Medical Association* 295, no. 20 (2006): 2341–2344.

4. K. Spiegel, R. Leproult, and E. Van Cauter, "Impact of Sleep Debt on Metabolic and Endocrine Function," *The Lancet* 354, no. 9188 (1999): 1435–1439.

5. Ibid.

6. H. Van Dongen, G. Maislin, J. Mullington, and D. Dinges, "The Cumulative Cost of Additional Wakefulness: Dose-response Effects on Neurobehavioral Functions and Sleep Physiology from Chronic Sleep Restriction and Total Sleep Deprivation," *Sleep* 26, no. 2 (2003): 117–126.

7. D. Dinges et al., "Cumulative Sleepiness, Mood Disturbance, and Psychomotor Vigilance Performance Decrements During a Week of Sleep Restricted to 4–5 Hours Per Night," *Sleep* 20, no. 4 (1997): 267–277.

8. L. Hunter, J. Rychnovsky, and S. Yount, "A Selective Review of Maternal Sleep Characteristics in the Postpartum Period," *Journal of Obstetric, Gynecologic, & Neonatal Nursing* 38, no. 1 (2009): 60–68.

9. D. Dinges et al., "Cumulative Sleepiness, Mood Disturbance,

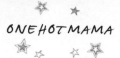
and Psychomotor Vigilance Performance Decrements During a Week of Sleep Restricted to 4–5 Hours Per Night," *Sleep* 20, no. 4 (1997): 267–277.

10. N. Isaacs, "Postnatal Yoga: Conditions and Cures for Both Mama and Babe," *Yoga Journal*, **www.yogajournal.com/lifestyle/1660.**

11. Legs-up-the-wall pose; Viparita Karani. *Yoga Journal*, **www.yogajournal.com/poses/690.**

Week Two

1. R. Reading and S. Reynolds, "Debt, Social Disadvantage, and Maternal Depression," *Social Science & Medicine* 53, no. 4 (2001): 441–453.

2. J. Pennebaker, *Opening Up: The Healing Power of Expressing Emotions* (New York: The Guilford Press, 1997).

3. M. Purcell, "The Health Benefits of Journaling," *Psych Central*, 2006, **http://psychcentral.com/lib/2006/the-health-benefits-of-journaling/.**

4. Ibid.

5. Ibid.

Week Three

1. National Research Council. *Weight Gain During Pregnancy: Reexamining the Guidelines.* Washington, DC: The National Academies Press (2009).

2. D. Benton and P. Parker, "Breakfast, Blood Glucose, and Cognition," *American Journal of Clinical Nutrition* 67 (1998): 772S–778S.

3. M. Oz, "Dr. Oz's Ultimate Supplement Checklist," *The Dr. Oz Show*, September 9 2010, **www.doctoroz.com/videos/dr-ozs-ultimate-supplement-checklist.**

4. Office of Dietary Supplements, "Dietary Supplement Fact

Sheet: Iron," National Institutes of Health, **http://ods
.od.nih.gov/factsheets/Iron-HealthProfessional/**.

5. M. Oz, "Dr. Oz's Ultimate Supplement Checklist," *The Dr. Oz
Show*, September 9 2010, **www.doctoroz.com/videos/
dr-ozs-ultimate-supplement-checklist**.

6. Ibid.

Week Four

1. National Center for Complementary and Alternative Medicine.
"Meditation for health purposes," **http://nccam.nih.gov/
health/meditation/overview.htm**.

2. E. R. Rosick. "Cortisol, Stress, and Health: Keeping levels of
the stress hormone cortisol in check may help prevent
illness and slow aging" *Life Extension Magazine*, December
2005, **www.lef.org/magazine/mag2005/dec2005_report_
cortisol_02.htm**.

3. B. K. Hölzel, J. Carmody, M. Vangel, C. Congleton, S. M.
Yerramsetti, T. Gard, S.W. Lazar. Mindfulness practice leads
to increases in regional brain gray matter density. *Psychiatry
Research: Neuroimaging* (2011) 191 (1): 36.

4. R. Wallace, M. Dillbeck, E. Jacobe, and B. Harrington, "The
Effects of the Transcendental Meditation and TM-Sidhi
Program on the Aging Process," *International Journal of
Neuroscience* 16, no. 1 (1982): 53–58.

5. P. J. O'Connor, N. P. Pronk, A. Tan, and R. P. Whitebird,
"Characteristics of adults who use prayer as an alternative
therapy." *Am. J. Health Promot.* (2005) 19:369–375.

Week Six

1. A. F. Shapiro, J. M. Gottman, S. Lubkin, R. Tyson, and C.
Swanson, "The Influence of the Marital Relationship
on Interactions Within the Mother-father-baby Triad"
(International Society for the Study of Behavioural
Development: Bern, 1998).

2. R. Epstein, "What Makes a Good Parent?" *Scientific American Mind*, November/December (2010): 46–51.

3. A. Simopoulos, "The Importance of the Ratio of Omega-6/Omega-3 Essential Fatty Acids," *Biomedical Pharmacotherapy* 56, no. 8 (2002): 365–379.

Week Seven

1. R. J. Johnson and T. Gower, *The Sugar Fix: The High-Fructose Fallout That Is Making You Fat and Sick* (New York: Pocket Books, 2008).

2. Centers for Disease Control and Prevention (CDC), "U.S. Obesity Trends" (2010).

3. N. Appleton, *Lick the Sugar Habit, Second Edition* (New York: Avery, 1996).

4. Associated Press, "Exercise Can Boost Mood of Depressed Patients" (January 23, 2006).

5. P. Salmon, "Effects of Physical Exercise on Anxiety, Depression, and Sensitivity to Stress: A Unifying Theory," *Clinical Psychology Review* 21, no. 1 (2001): 33–61.

Week Eight

1. A. Meltzoff, "Born to Learn: What Infants Learn from Watching Us," in *The Role of Early Experience in Infant Development*, eds. N. Fox & J. G. Worhol (Skillman, New Jersey: Pediatric Institute Publications, 1999).

2. C. Weaver, "Health Benefits of Coffee," *EzineArticles.com*, January 24, 2007, **http://EzineArticles.com/430304**.

3. Ibid.

4. M. Eskelinen, T. Ngandu, J. Tuomilehto, H. Soininen, and M. Kivipelto, "Midlife Coffee and Tea Drinking and the Risk of Late-life Dementia: A Population-based CAIDE Study," *Journal of Alzheimer's Disease* 16, no. 1 (2009): 85–91.

5. K.M. Zelman. "The Buzz on Coffee: The latest research shows your morning pick-me-up may be brimming with health

benefits." WebMD, May 7, 2008, **www.webmd.com/diet/features/the-buzz-on-coffee.**

6. C. Berlin, H. Denson, C. Daniel, and R. Ward, "Disposition of Dietary Caffeine in Milk, Saliva, and Plasma of Lactating Women," *Pediatrics* 73, no. 1 (1984): 59–63.

Week Nine

1. "Mayo Clinic Study Finds Optimists Report a Higher Quality of Life Than Pessimists," *Science Daily* (August 13, 2002).

2. Ibid.

3. Ibid.

4. Ibid.

5. D. Snowdon, *Aging with Grace: What the Nun Study Teaches Us About Leading Longer, Healthier, and More Meaningful Lives* (New York: Bantam, 2001).

6. J. Gottman and R. Levenson, "What Predicts Change in Marital Interaction Over Time? A Study of Alternative Models," *Family Process* 38, no. 2 (1999).

7. K. Zelman, "Five Ways to Keep from Overloading on Calories When You Have an Alcoholic Drink," WebMD, 2011, **www .webmd.com/diet/features/low-calorie-cocktails.**

8. K. Zelman, "Best and Worst Appetizers," WebMD, May 9, 2011, **www.webmd.com/diet/ss/slideshow-best-and-worst-appetizers.**

Week Ten

1. C. Manske, C. Lorincz, and R. Zernicke, "Bone Health: Part 2, Physical Activity," *Sports Health: A Multidisciplinary Approach 1,* no. 4 (July/August 2009): 341–346.

Week Twelve

1. J. O'Doherty, J. Winston, H. Critchley, D. Perrett, D. Burt, and R. Dolan, "Beauty in a Smile: The Role of

Medial Orbitofrontal Cortex in Facial Attractiveness,"
Neuropsychologia 41, no. 2 (2003): 147–155.

2. I. Lee, L. Djoussé, H. Sesso, L. Wang, and J. Buring, "Physical
Activity and Weight Gain Prevention," *The Journal of the
American Medical Association* 303, no. 12 (2010): 1173–1179.

★ ◻ ★

ACKNOWLEDGMENTS

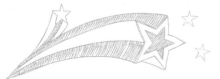

First of all, I would like to thank my greatest love and partner for life, Steve Cox, who has made so many things possible. He has always challenged me to be the very best I possibly can and has been my ever-supportive partner through this entire process. He is also the best father I could have chosen for our three precious children.

I would like to acknowledge my precious daughters, Ella and Elena, and my sweet son, Kellan. They have tolerated a mom who is on her computer for hours each day. My children give me daily inspiration and keep me smiling!

I would also like to thank my loving and encouraging parents, Gene and Cindy Day, who have always believed in me, as well as my brother, Brian, and my entire fabulous family. My mom and my mother-in-law, Susan Cox, have been reading and editing my work for years, and my father-in-law, Ed, has supported me with love as my business coach.

My fabulous exercise models, Anne Rylance, Tyanne Luken, Leah Crouser, and Laura Larson, have been dear friends for many years and have always offered me their love and encouragement. In addition, they have motivated me with the way they manage their lives and stay so fit as mothers. I also want to give a shout-out to all of my beloved girlfriends from Watertown, South Dakota, as well as from college and graduate school, and to my family-like military friends who live all over the world. You all know who you are, and please know how much I love you and have been inspired by each of you!

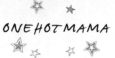

ONE HOT MAMA

Finally, I would like to thank Hay House for supporting me and working with me on this important project, as well as my wonderful and detailed editors, Brookes Nohlgren and Lisa Bernier, who helped bring this book to life.

★ ◻ ★

ABOUT THE AUTHOR

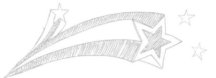

Erin Cox is a personal-development author, motivational speaker, wellness coach, and mother of three who advises women on how to live more balanced, joyful, and healthy lives. Erin has become an expert in leading a balanced, healthy, fulfilled life as a mother through her personal experiences since delivering her first child in 2006. As the wife of an Air Force F-15 pilot, Erin has moved four times since her wedding in 2002, and as a result she has bonded with and learned from mothers from all over the world. Erin loves to hang out with her husband, play with her children, run, hike, do yoga, cook, and of course, write! Erin has also worked in water resources science and engineering. She received her BS in biology from North Dakota State University and an MS in water resources from the Civil Engineering Department at the University of Minnesota.

Erin believes wholeheartedly that motherhood is one of the most beautiful blessings that life has to offer, but it also presents a multitude of additional challenges for self-care and personal development. Erin's mission is to love, nurture, and support women so they can love and feel good about themselves, live their dream lives, and offer their best selves to their loved ones.

Connect with Erin at **www.erincox.com**.

★☐★

We hope you enjoyed this Hay House book. If you'd like to receive our online catalog featuring additional information on Hay House books and products, or if you'd like to find out more about the Hay Foundation, please contact:

Hay House, Inc., P.O. Box 5100, Carlsbad, CA 92018-5100
(760) 431-7695 or (800) 654-5126
(760) 431-6948 (fax) or (800) 650-5115 (fax)
www.hayhouse.com® • **www.hayfoundation.org**

Published and distributed in Australia by: Hay House Australia Pty. Ltd., 18/36 Ralph St., Alexandria NSW 2015 • *Phone:* 612-9669-4299 *Fax:* 612-9669-4144 • www.hayhouse.com.au

Published and distributed in the United Kingdom by: Hay House UK, Ltd., 292B Kensal Rd., London W10 5BE • *Phone:* 44-20-8962-1230 *Fax:* 44-20-8962-1239 • www.hayhouse.co.uk

Published and distributed in the Republic of South Africa by: Hay House SA (Pty), Ltd., P.O. Box 990, Witkoppen 2068 • *Phone/Fax:* 27-11-467-8904 www.hayhouse.co.za

Published in India by: Hay House Publishers India, Muskaan Complex, Plot No. 3, B-2, Vasant Kunj, New Delhi 110 070 • *Phone:* 91-11-4176-1620 *Fax:* 91-11-4176-1630 • www.hayhouse.co.in

Distributed in Canada by: Raincoast, 9050 Shaughnessy St., Vancouver, B.C. V6P 6E5 • *Phone:* (604) 323-7100 • *Fax:* (604) 323-2600 • www.raincoast.com

Take Your Soul on a Vacation

Visit **www.HealYourLife.com®** to regroup, recharge, and reconnect with your own magnificence.Featuring blogs, mind-body-spirit news, and life-changing wisdom from Louise Hay and friends.

Visit **www.HealYourLife.com** today!